Elevating Egg Quality

Proven Strategies for Fertility and Successful IVF

By

Melissa W. Giblin

Copyright

Disclaimer

This book serves as informative support, not medical counsel. Melissa W. Giblin, the author, is not a medical professional. Readers are advised to consult medical professionals for tailored guidance. The content's general nature may not apply universally, and individual results may differ. Any specific medical procedures discussed are for informational purposes, not endorsements. While efforts ensure accuracy, the author disclaims responsibility for errors. Readers assume responsibility for their decisions and release the author from any claims arising from book use. Prioritize personal health; seek professional advice for personalized care.

Table of Content

INTRODUCTION

Understanding Fertility Challenges

The journey to motherhood is a very personal and frequently challenging endeavor. Many people are filled with excitement, anticipation, and great hopes when they dream of starting a family. However, a considerable number of couples encounter unforeseen setbacks along the way. The purpose of this article is to provide an in-depth overview of the reproductive issues that people and couples may face, shedding light on the complex web of circumstances that might influence the capacity to conceive.

Fertility's Difficulty

Fertility, defined as the ability to conceive and carry a pregnancy to term, is a delicate balance of biological, environmental, and behavioral factors. While some people are fortunate to have a quick and painless path to parenting, others have a more difficult and emotionally exhausting process. Understanding the elements that contribute to reproductive issues is critical for people who are navigating this treacherous terrain.

Factors of Biology

The complex structures of the reproductive system are one of the key factors of fertility. The menstrual cycle, hormonal balance, and ovarian health are all important factors for women. Conditions such as polycystic ovarian syndrome (PCOS) or endometriosis can have an influence on fertility, posing challenges that must be carefully navigated. Fertility can be influenced by male factors such as sperm count, motility, and morphology, making it a shared duty for couples.

Influences of Lifestyle and Environment

Aside from biology, lifestyle choices and environmental influences can also have a substantial impact on fertility. The modern way of life is typically associated with high levels of stress, inconsistent sleep patterns, and improper dietary habits, all of which can contribute to fertility issues. Toxins found in daily items and contaminants may also play a role, emphasizing the necessity of fostering a fertile environment.

Nutrition and Its Function

The adage "you are what you eat" is especially true when it comes to fertility. Nutrition is important for both men and women's reproductive health. A well-balanced, nutrient-dense diet promotes hormonal balance, egg and sperm quality, and overall reproductive function. Poor food choices, on the other hand, might contribute to fertility troubles, stressing the need of mindful nutrition on the route to parenting.

The Relationship Between Age and Fertility

When it comes to fertility issues, age is an important aspect. Women's fertility naturally declines as they age, with the greatest dramatic reduction occurring in their late 30s and early 40s. Age can also effect male fertility, albeit to a lesser amount. Understanding the effect of age on fertility is critical for people and couples who want to start a family.

Managing Emotional Stress

The emotional cost of fertility issues should not be underestimated. For those facing challenges, the pleasure and expectation that frequently accompany the decision to have a child can quickly turn into frustration, despair, and even grief. Open communication, support networks, and seeking professional help can all help you navigate the emotional pressure that typically comes with the quest for parenting.

Looking for Answers: Medical Interventions and Beyond

Individuals and couples who are facing fertility issues have options. Medical science advancements have paved the door for a variety of interventions, ranging from fertility treatments like in vitro fertilization (IVF) to assisted reproductive technologies. These approaches, however, are not universal, and the decision to explore medical measures is deeply personal.

Holistic approaches to fertility are gaining favor in addition to conventional therapies. Stress reduction, regular exercise, and following a fertility-friendly diet are all becoming essential components of reproductive care. Integrative techniques that incorporate the full person—mind, body, and spirit—are becoming increasingly valued in resolving fertility issues.

The journey to motherhood, while frequently difficult, demonstrates the perseverance and determination of individuals and couples attempting to start a family. Understanding the complexities of reproductive issues is the first step toward making informed decisions and making empowered choices. As we explore the nuances of fertility, let us take a caring and supportive attitude, acknowledging that each road to parenting is unique and deserves to be respected. In doing so, we contribute to a more inclusive and understanding debate about fertility, developing a community where the dream of starting a family is met with empathy, encouragement, and steadfast support.

The Importance of Lifestyle and Nutrition

As individuals and couples negotiate this path, one aspect of reproductive health emerges as a constant: the junction of lifestyle and diet. In this article, we will look at the fundamental importance of these aspects in the context of fertility, delving into the nuanced ways in which the decisions we make in our everyday lives, from the food we consume to how we deal with stress, can have a substantial impact on our ability to conceive and nurture life.

Recognizing the Holistic Approach

At its root, fertility is a holistic idea that extends beyond the physical act of conception. It includes both couples' overall health and well-being, including physical, emotional, and even environmental variables. Recognizing the holistic nature of fertility leads us to investigate how lifestyle and diet play a role in this complicated tapestry.

The Foundation for Nutrition

Nutrition is a critical component in the quest for fertility. The foods we eat supply the building blocks for our bodies, regulating hormone balance, reproductive organ health, and general reproductive system functionality. A well-balanced, nutrient-dense diet not only supports the body's fundamental functions but also plays an important role in producing an environment suitable for conception.

Dietary Influence on Reproductive Hormones

Important reproductive hormones like estrogen and progesterone in women and testosterone in men are inextricably related to the meals we eat. Zinc, vitamin D, and omega-3 fatty acids all play important roles in hormone regulation. Zinc, for example, is required for testosterone production in men, whereas optimal vitamin D levels are connected with enhanced fertility in both men and women. Understanding the complex interplay between nutrition and hormonal balance is essential for improving fertility.

Fertility-Friendly Nutrients and Foods

Specific nutrients and meals have been identified as having a good impact on fertility. Antioxidants present in fruits and vegetables aid in the fight against oxidative stress, which can harm reproductive health. Folate, which can be found in leafy greens and legumes, is essential for preventing neural tube abnormalities in early pregnancy. Omega-3 fatty acids, found in fish and flaxseeds, help with reproductive health.

Avoiding Negative Dietary Patterns

It is also critical to be mindful of food trends that may interfere with fertility. Consumption of processed meals, sugary beverages, and trans fats has been linked to fertility problems. These inflammatory food choices can disturb hormonal balance and contribute to illnesses like insulin resistance, which can have an influence on fertility.

The Influence of Lifestyle Decisions

Along with nutrition, lifestyle decisions have a significant impact on fertility. The current pace of life frequently involves high levels of stress, inconsistent sleep patterns, and sedentary activities, all of which can lead to fertility issues.

Recognizing the interdependence of lifestyle factors is critical for those looking to improve their reproductive health.

Stress Reduction

Stress, which is all too common in today's fast-paced society, can have a negative impact on fertility. The body's stress response, which is essential for survival, can have an unintended impact on reproductive function. Chronic stress can cause menstrual cycle disruption in women and sperm quality in males. Incorporating stress-reduction strategies such as mindfulness, yoga, or meditation becomes not only a way to improve overall well-being but also a critical component of reproductive care.

Fertility and Exercise

Regular physical activity is essential for a healthy lifestyle, but excessive exercise might have an adverse effect on fertility. Intense, persistent exercise can disrupt women's menstrual cycles and have an impact on men's sperm production. Maintaining a healthy balance through moderate exercise benefits general health and may have a good impact on fertility.

The Function of Sleep

In discussions regarding fertility, quality sleep is sometimes overlooked. Sleep disruptions can disrupt hormonal homeostasis, altering reproductive hormones. Creating a sleep-friendly atmosphere and practicing healthy sleeping habits can improve both general health and fertility.

Fertility and Environmental Factors

Fertility is also affected by the environment in which we live, work, and breathe. Toxins in the environment, both inside and outside our houses, can have an impact on reproductive health. Understanding and minimizing environmental impacts is critical to maximizing fertility, from endocrine-disrupting chemicals in common items to contaminants in the air we breathe.

Toxins in Commonplace Products

Chemicals in common household products, ranging from cleaning supplies to personal care items, might disturb hormonal balance. Phthalates, which can be found in plastics and personal care items, are known endocrine disruptors. Choosing "phthalate-free" products and natural alternatives can help prevent exposure to these potentially dangerous compounds.

Making Your Environment Fertility-Friendly

Mindful choices in the home environment can help to optimize fertility. This involves limiting pesticide exposure, eating organic foods if possible, and being mindful of air quality. Small modifications, like as utilizing non-toxic cleaning products and decreasing plastic use, help to create a fertility-friendly environment.

Fertility Options That Are Empowering

Individuals and couples are not passive bystanders in the face of these factors; they are empowered decision-makers with the ability to influence their reproductive health. Adopting a proactive strategy that includes informed food choices, mindful lifestyle behaviors, and environmental awareness builds a solid foundation for fertility enhancement.

The Importance of Prenatal Care

Preconception care, or a proactive approach to health before pregnancy, has gained popularity in fertility debates. Prior to attempting conception, it is necessary to optimize health by nutrition, lifestyle, and medical measures. This proactive strategy tries to address potential reproductive issues before they become major roadblocks.

Seeking Professional Help

Each individual and couple's path to motherhood is unique. Seeking professional advice from healthcare providers, dietitians, and fertility specialists can provide tailored insights and assistance. When medical interventions are required, they can be approached cooperatively, with a focus on holistic care that takes into account the individual's total well-being.

Life is Nurtured from Within

The threads of lifestyle and diet are woven with care and intention into the complicated fabric of fertility. Recognizing the importance of these factors enables individuals and couples to take proactive efforts toward improving their reproductive health. Every decision we make, from the meals we eat to fuel our bodies to the everyday decisions that shape our lives, has the ability to grow life from inside. Let us navigate this journey with informed choices, compassion for ourselves and others, and an unwavering belief in the possibility of creating life—a journey that begins with a profound recognition of the importance of lifestyle and nutrition.

CHAPTER 1

Female Reproductive System

A Comprehensive Guide

The female reproductive system is a biological engineering marvel, orchestrating a complicated ballet of hormones, organs, and processes to permit the incredible journey of conception and pregnancy. In this post, we will take a complete look at the female reproductive system, delving into its anatomy, functioning, and the complexities that make it such an important part of human life.

Female Reproductive System Anatomy

A symphony of organs plays a unique function in the delicate process of reproduction at the center of the female reproductive system. The ovaries, fallopian tubes, uterus, and vagina are the major components.

The Ovum Factories are the ovaries.

The ovaries, like hard working factories, are in charge of manufacturing eggs, or ovum, and reproductive hormones. These almond-sized organs, located on either side of the uterus, contain thousands of follicles, each holding an immature egg. Ovulation, or the release of a mature egg, happens about once a month, marking a critical stage in the menstrual cycle.

Fallopian Tubes: Conception Conduits

The fallopian tubes are fragile tubes that connect the ovaries to the uterus. Fertilization occurs within these short tubes. Following ovulation, the released egg travels through the fallopian tubes. If sperm is available and fertilizes the egg successfully during this transit, the resulting fertilized egg, or zygote, continues its migration towards the uterus for implantation.

The Uterus as a Nurturing Chamber

The uterus, a muscular organ that resembles an inverted pear, is the focal point of pregnancy. The endometrium, the inner lining, thickens in preparation for a prospective embryo. If fertilization takes place, the embryo attaches into the endometrium, kicking off the remarkable process of pregnancy. The endometrial lining is lost during menstruation if fertilization does not occur.

Cervix: The Doorway to the Uterus

The cervix, or bottom section of the uterus, serves as a connection point between the uterus and the vagina. This cylindrical channel allows menstrual blood to flow freely and serves as a sperm entry point during intercourse. The cervix is important in birthing because it dilates to allow the baby to pass from the uterus to the vagina.

Birth Canal and Other Information

The vagina, also known as the birth canal, is a muscular tube that connects the cervix to the external genitalia. The vagina also serves as a receptacle for the penis during sexual intercourse, in addition to its role in birthing. It is a dynamic organ that may extend to meet a variety of activities, including sexual intimacy, menstrual blood flow, and birthing.

The Menstrual Cycle: A Hormone Symphony

The menstrual cycle, a periodic interplay of hormones directing the preparation for prospective pregnancy, is important to the female reproductive system. The menstrual cycle lasts about 28 days on average, however deviations are normal.

Shedding and Renewal During the Menstrual Cycle

The cycle begins with the menstrual phase, which is distinguished by the shedding of the uterine lining. Menstruation, often known as the menstrual period, usually lasts 3 to 7 days. At the same time, the ovaries begin to prepare a new cohort of follicles for possible ovulation.

Ovulation is on the way during the Follicular Phase.

The follicular phase begins after menstruation, when the pituitary gland secretes follicle-stimulating hormone (FSH). This hormone causes the ovaries to produce a cluster of follicles, with one becoming the dominant follicle. The dominant follicle releases estrogen as it matures, preparing the uterine lining for a prospective embryo.

The Ovulatory Phase: The Fertility Peak

Ovulation is triggered by a rise in luteinizing hormone (LH) midway through the cycle. When the mature follicle ruptures, the egg is released into the fallopian tube. This is the most fertile period, with a window of opportunity for conception. If fertilization has place, the zygote continues its journey to the uterus.

Preparing for Pregnancy or Menstruation During the Luteal Phase

Following ovulation, the luteal phase occurs, during which the burst follicle converts into the corpus luteum. This structure produces progesterone, which helps to maintain the uterine lining in preparation for a possible pregnancy. In the absence of fertilization, the corpus luteum disintegrates, resulting in a decline in hormonal support and the commencement of menstruation.

Estrogen and progesterone are hormonal players.

In controlling the female reproductive system, two important hormones, estrogen and progesterone, take center stage. These hormones, which are predominantly produced by the ovaries, have a significant impact on the menstrual cycle and other reproductive processes.

Estrogen: The Growth Engineer

Estrogen, which is produced by growing follicles in the ovaries, is a versatile hormone with a wide range of actions. It promotes an environment conducive to embryo implantation by stimulating the thickness of the uterine lining during the follicular phase. In addition to its reproductive function, estrogen affects bone density, cardiovascular health, and even mood.

Maintaining the Uterine Environment with Progesterone

During the luteal phase, progesterone is secreted by the corpus luteum and works in tandem with estrogen. It preserves the uterine lining's integrity, preparing it to support a prospective pregnancy. Progesterone is also involved in breast development and menstrual cycle management.

Disorders and Difficulties

While the female reproductive system is an engineering marvel, it is not immune to illnesses and obstacles. Several disorders can have an effect on fertility and reproductive health, demanding knowledge and, in some circumstances, medical intervention.

PCOS (Polycystic Ovary Syndrome): A Hormonal Imbalance

PCOS is a common endocrine illness marked by a hormonal imbalance in the reproductive system. It can cause irregular menstrual cycles, ovarian cysts, and ovulation problems. Women with PCOS may have difficulty conceiving and are more likely to develop illnesses such as type 2 diabetes.

Endometriosis: Tissue Other Than the Uterus

Endometriosis is a condition in which tissue that resembles the uterine lining grows outside of the uterus. This aberrant tissue reacts to hormonal fluctuations by generating inflammation, discomfort, and adhesion formation. Endometriosis can impair fertility by interfering with the function of the ovaries and fallopian tubes.

Noncancerous Growth of Uterine Fibroids

Uterine fibroids are noncancerous growths that form within the uterine walls. While these growths are usually harmless, they can cause symptoms such as heavy menstrual bleeding, pelvic pain, and pressure. Fibroids can interfere with conception and pregnancy depending on their size and location.

Education and Advocacy for Reproductive Health

Understanding the complexities of the female reproductive system is a valuable tool for individuals and couples embarking on the journey of conception. Individuals are empowered by education to make educated decisions about their reproductive health and to seek timely medical assistance when necessary. Beyond personal empowerment, societal advocacy for reproductive health education helps to a society that recognizes and supports individuals' various reproductive paths.

Celebrating Life's Complexity

The female reproductive system is fundamental and awe-inspiring in the magnificent tapestry of life. Each component illustrates the intricate architecture that sustains the continuation of human existence, from the microscopic dance of hormones to the macroscopic processes of conception and birthing. We can develop a culture that values and embraces the diversity of reproductive experiences by unlocking the secrets of the female reproductive system.

Insights about the Menstrual Cycle

A crucial element of the female reproductive system is the menstrual cycle, a monthly symphony of hormonal swings and physiological changes. The menstrual cycle provides important insights into overall health and well-being in addition to its role in signaling fertility. This investigation delves into the many components of the menstrual cycle, revealing the subtleties that define this delicate biological rhythm.

A Monthly Symphony for Understanding the Menstrual Cycle

The menstrual cycle is, at its core, a periodic sequence of events choreographed by the delicate interaction of hormones that prepares the female body for the possibility of conception. The menstrual cycle is divided into various phases, each with its own distinctive characteristics and functions, and lasts an average of 28 days, however individual variances are typical.

Menstruation: Mother Nature's Reset Button

The cycle starts with the menstrual phase, which is characterized by the shedding of the uterine lining, also known as menstruation. This phase normally lasts 3 to 7 days and marks the beginning of a new cycle. Concurrently, the ovaries begin to generate a new cohort of follicles in preparation for potential ovulation.

Follicular Phase: A Growth Symphony

The follicular phase begins after menstruation, when the pituitary gland secretes follicle-stimulating hormone (FSH). This hormone causes the ovaries to produce a cluster of follicles, each containing an immature egg. As these follicles mature, estrogen is released, which aids in the preparation of the uterine lining for a prospective embryo.

The Fertile Window During the Ovulatory Phase

A rise in luteinizing hormone (LH) midway through the cycle causes ovulation, or the release of a mature egg from the dominant follicle. As the egg begins its trip in the fallopian tube, it reaches the height of fertility. The ovulatory phase, which lasts from 24 to 48 hours, provides a small yet critical window for conception.

Luteal Stage: Getting Ready for Pregnancy or Menstruation

The luteal phase begins after ovulation. The burst follicle converts into the corpus luteum, which releases progesterone. This hormone maintains the uterine lining, allowing embryo implantation to occur. In the absence of fertilization, the corpus luteum disintegrates, resulting in a decline in hormonal support and the commencement of menstruation.

Estrogen and Progesterone Lead the Hormonal Orchestra

The hormonal players, estrogen and progesterone, which are largely produced by the ovaries, are crucial to the menstrual cycle. These hormones have a significant impact on the various stages of the cycle, coordinating the delicate dance of reproductive activities.

Estrogen: The Growth Engineer

During the follicular phase, the versatile hormone estrogen takes center stage. Estrogen, which is produced by growing follicles in the ovaries, encourages the thickening of the uterine lining, producing an environment favorable for embryo implantation. In addition to its reproductive function, estrogen affects bone density, cardiovascular health, and even mood.

Maintaining the Uterine Environment with Progesterone

Progesterone is secreted by the corpus luteum during the luteal phase. This hormone works in tandem with estrogen to preserve the uterine lining's integrity and prepare it to sustain a prospective pregnancy. Progesterone is also involved in breast development and menstrual cycle management.

Fertility Insights: Decoding the Menstrual Calendar

Understanding the menstrual cycle can help you become more fertile. The fertile window, which occurs around ovulation, provides an excellent possibility for conception. Individuals and couples can identify this window and enhance their chances of conception by tracking menstrual cycles using methods such as recording basal body temperature, monitoring cervical mucus changes, or utilizing ovulation predictor kits.

Menstrual irregularities: Signs of Poor Health?

Menstrual cycle irregularities, such as irregular cycles, nonexistent menstruation (amenorrhea), or extremely severe bleeding (menorrhagia), might be indicators of underlying health issues.

Menstrual irregularities may indicate the presence of conditions such as polycystic ovarian syndrome (PCOS), thyroid issues, or hormonal imbalances, necessitating additional examination and medical intervention.

The Influence of Lifestyle on the Menstrual Cycle

Lifestyle decisions have a significant impact on the menstrual cycle. Stress, food, and exercise can all have an impact on hormonal balance and general reproductive health, underscoring the link between lifestyle and monthly rhythm.

Menstrual Health and Stress

The complex association between stress and the menstrual cycle is widely known. Chronic stress can upset the delicate hormonal balance, resulting in irregular periods or even amenorrhea. Stress management approaches, such as mindfulness, meditation, and relaxation exercises, have the ability to restore menstrual cycle equilibrium.

Dietary Factors Affecting Menstrual Health

Nutrition is critical to hormone balance and reproductive health. Adequate intake of key nutrients such as iron, B vitamins, and omega-3 fatty acids promotes the reproductive system's general health. Diets deficient in vital nutrients or characterized by extreme calorie restriction, on the other hand, may contribute to menstrual abnormalities.

Menstrual Regularity and Exercise

Regular physical activity is an essential component of a healthy lifestyle, but excessive exercise might have an impact on menstruation regularity. Exercise can cause amenorrhea or irregular cycles, a condition known as exercise-induced hypothalamic amenorrhea. Striking a balance through modest exercise benefits general health without interfering with menstruation regularity.

Common Menstrual Disorders: Overcoming Obstacles

While the menstrual cycle usually works as a well-coordinated symphony, certain illnesses and ailments can throw off the rhythm. To ensure optimal reproductive health, it is critical to recognize and manage these issues.

Dysmenorrhea: The Struggle with Painful Periods

Dysmenorrhea, often known as painful menstruation, is a frequent menstrual disease that can have a negative influence on one's quality of life. It may be linked to illnesses like endometriosis or uterine fibroids. Pain treatment drugs, hormonal therapy, and lifestyle changes are examples of management options.

Premenstrual Syndrome (PMS): A Regular Visitor

PMS refers to a group of physical and mental symptoms that occur in the days preceding menstruation. Mood swings, bloating, and breast tenderness are all possible symptoms. PMS symptoms are frequently treated with lifestyle changes, food adjustments, and pharmaceuticals.

Menarche Celebration: A Rite of Passage

Menarche, or the beginning of menstruation, is an important rite of passage in a woman's life. Menarche has cultural, social, and psychological significance aside from its biological ramifications. Menarche-related open interactions and supportive surroundings contribute to happy menstruation experiences and develop a healthy relationship with one's reproductive health.

Accepting Life's Cyclical Nature

We get a profound grasp of reproductive health as well as an appreciation for the cyclical essence of life itself by deciphering the nuances of the menstrual cycle. The monthly ebb and flow of hormones, the delicate ballet of physiological processes, and the potential for life development highlight the female reproductive system's miracle. As we accept the menstrual cycle's cyclical nature, let us cultivate a society that celebrates and supports individuals' unique experiences, recognizing the tremendous wisdom embedded within this delicate biological

pattern.

CHAPTER 2

The Effect of Diet on Fertility

Reproductive Wellness Nutritional Guidelines

A fertility-friendly diet starts with a foundation based on balance and diversity. Nutrient-rich diets are vital for reproductive health, since they maintain hormonal balance and provide an environment conducive to conception.

Including a Variety of Vegetables and Fruits

Dive into a rainbow of colorful veggies and fruits, each with its own set of vitamins, minerals, and antioxidants. Including a variety of fruits and vegetables ensures a varied spectrum of nutrients that contribute to general health and fertility. Nature's bounty provides a multitude of fertility-nurturing options, ranging from folate-rich leafy greens to antioxidant-rich berries.

Choosing Whole Grains for Long-Term Energy

Whole grains like quinoa, brown rice, and oats are essential components of a fertility-focused diet. These grains include complex carbs that slowly release energy, maintaining stable blood sugar levels. Stable blood sugar levels are necessary for hormonal balance, which is a critical aspect in regulating fertility. To maximize nutritional benefits, choose whole grains over refined grains.

Protein Power: Reproductive Health Protein Sources

Protein is an essential component of a fertility-friendly diet, as it aids in the formation and repair of tissues. Choose high-quality sources including lean meats, poultry, fish, and eggs, as well as plant-based options like legumes and nuts. These protein sources are high in amino acids and vital nutrients, which help the body's reproductive activities.

Hormonal Balance and Healthy Fats

To maintain hormonal balance, include healthy fats in your diet such as avocados, nuts, seeds, and olive oil. Omega-3 fatty acids, present in fatty fish such as salmon and flaxseeds, are essential for reproductive health. These lipids help to regulate hormones and develop a healthy uterine lining, creating an ideal environment for conception.

Fertility-Related Nutrients

Investigating the details of critical nutrients reveals the major players who have a direct impact on reproductive health. These nutrients, which range from antioxidants to vitamins and minerals, are critical in promoting fertility.

Folate: An Important Preconception Nutrient

Folate, a B-vitamin, plays an important role in preconception care. Adequate folate intake promotes neural tube development in the early stages of pregnancy, lowering the chance of neural tube abnormalities. Folate is abundant in leafy greens, fortified cereals, and legumes, underscoring the relevance of this nutrient in preconception planning.

Iron: An Energy and Oxygen Transporter

Iron is a super vitamin that helps with energy levels and oxygen delivery throughout the body. Maintaining adequate iron levels is critical for women of reproductive age because iron shortage can lead to anemia, which can influence fertility. Iron consumption is increased in a fertility-focused diet by eating lean meats, lentils, spinach, and fortified cereals.

Calcium: Laying Firm Foundations

Calcium contributes to bone health while also impacting reproductive function in reproductive health. Calcium is found in dairy products, fortified plant-based milk, and leafy greens. Getting enough calcium is especially important for women who are considering a pregnancy because it helps the developing fetus develop a healthy skeletal structure.

Zinc: Promoting Male and Female Fertility

Zinc is a trace mineral important for both male and female reproductive health. Zinc is essential for sperm production in males and egg development and fertilization in women. Zinc-rich foods such as oysters, pumpkin seeds, and chickpeas should be included in your diet to provide adequate quantities of this fertility-supporting mineral.

Dietary Choices and Lifestyle Factors

Aside from individual nutrients, lifestyle variables and overall dietary patterns all contribute to the overall picture of reproductive fitness. Considering these larger variables improves the efficiency of fertility nutritional guidelines.

Hydration: The Unsung Reproductive Wellness Hero

The role of water in reproductive health should not be disregarded in the midst of the focus on specific nutrients. Staying hydrated benefits all physical systems, including those important for conception. Water is required to sustain cervical mucus, a material that helps sperm reach the egg. A healthy uterine lining and adequate blood flow to reproductive organs are also supported by adequate hydration.

Moderation: Finding a Healthy Balance in Your Diet

While fertility-friendly foods are vital, it's also important to approach dietary choices with a temperance perspective. Aim for a healthy mix of carbs, proteins, and fats, avoiding extremes that can disturb hormonal equilibrium. An overly restrictive diet might result in nutritional deficits, which can have an influence on reproductive health.

Caffeine and Alcohol: Consumption with Caution

Caffeine and alcohol should be consumed in moderation. While moderate caffeine usage is generally seen as harmless, high caffeine consumption has been associated to fertility problems. Similarly, excessive alcohol use can disturb hormonal balance and have an effect on fertility. Adopting attentive and moderate use of these substances is consistent with the larger goal of promoting reproductive health.

Individualized Fertility Nutrition Approaches

Recognizing the individuality of each person's physiology and lifestyle, it becomes clear that a one-size-fits-all approach to reproductive diet may not be optimum. Nutritional guidelines are more successful when they are tailored to individual needs, tastes, and any underlying conditions.

Consultation with Medical Professionals

Seeking advice from healthcare professionals, such as dietitians and fertility specialists, is essential in developing a personalized strategy to fertility nutrition. Preexisting health issues, specialized nutritional demands, and lifestyle concerns are all variables in personalized guidance. This coordinated approach ensures that food choices are consistent with both reproductive goals and overall health.

Paying Attention to the Body's Signals

The body frequently sends messages and indications about its nutritional requirements. Tuning in to these signals is practicing mindful eating and paying attention to how the body reacts to various foods. Sensitivities or intolerances can have an impact on reproductive health, and being aware of these subtleties allows for modifications that benefit general well-being.

Fertility Enhancement Through Nutritional Knowledge

Nutritional guidelines emerge as strong tools for developing reproductive wellness as individuals and couples negotiate the complex landscape of fertility. A fertility-friendly diet rich in variety and nutrient-dense foods sets the foundation for hormonal balance, healthy reproductive function, and the establishment of a fertile environment. Individuals can begin on a journey that corresponds with the profound knowledge embedded within the delicate dance of fertility by accepting these dietary truths and weaving them into the fabric of daily life.

Conception and Reproductive Wellness Foods

Understanding the impact of nutrition on fertility allows for more deliberate food choices that promote reproductive health. In this detailed guide, we look at which foods to eat and which to avoid, offering a road map for individuals and couples looking to improve their fertility.

Fertility Foods to Include

The Rainbow Palette of Colorful Vegetables and Fruits

Accept the colorful spectrum of veggies and fruits, with each color signifying a distinct collection of nutrients and antioxidants. Folate, a B-vitamin essential for early pregnancy, is found in leafy greens such as spinach and kale. Berries, which are high in antioxidants, fight oxidative stress and promote reproductive health.

Whole Grains: The Building Blocks of Long-Term Energy

To get complex carbs, choose whole grains like quinoa, brown rice, and oats. These grains gradually release energy, assisting in the maintenance of steady blood sugar levels. Stable blood sugar levels are necessary for hormonal balance, which is a critical aspect in regulating fertility.

Lean Proteins: Reproductive Tissue Building Blocks

Prioritize lean protein sources such as poultry, fish, and eggs, as well as plant-based options like legumes and nuts. Proteins are required for the formation and repair of tissues, particularly those important for reproductive health. A diversified amino acid composition is ensured by incorporating a variety of protein sources.

Hormonal Balance with Healthy Fats

Consume healthy fats from avocados, nuts, seeds, and olive oil. Omega-3 fatty acids, present in fatty fish such as salmon and flaxseeds, help to regulate hormones and develop a healthy uterine lining. These lipids are critical in generating an ideal environment for conception.

Foods High in Folate: Beneficial for Early Pregnancy

Prioritize foods high in folate, a B vitamin important for neural tube development in early pregnancy. Folate is abundant in leafy greens, lentils, fortified cereals, and citrus fruits.

Adequate folate intake is especially crucial for those planning to become pregnant.

Iron-Rich Options for Energy and Oxygen Transport

Iron-rich foods should be included to help with energy levels and oxygen delivery throughout the body. Iron is found in lean meats, lentils, spinach, and fortified cereals. Maintaining optimal iron levels is critical for reproductive health, since it helps to prevent disorders such as anemia.

Calcium for Bone Health and Other Purposes

Make calcium-rich diets a priority for bone health and reproductive function. Calcium consumption is increased by dairy products, fortified plant-based milk, and leafy greens. Calcium is vital for women of reproductive age because it supports bone health as well as reproductive processes.

Choices for Increasing Zinc: Promoting Reproductive Health

Include zinc-rich foods, which are essential for both male and female reproductive health. Zinc is abundant in oysters, pumpkin seeds, chickpeas, and lean meats. Maintaining enough zinc levels aids sperm production in men and egg development in women.

Hydration: The Unsung Reproductive Wellness Hero

Maintain adequate hydration to maintain overall biological functions, especially those essential for reproduction. Water is necessary for the maintenance of cervical mucus, which aids sperm in reaching the egg. A healthy uterine lining and adequate blood flow to reproductive organs are also supported by adequate hydration.

Caffeine and alcohol should be consumed in moderation.

Caffeine and alcohol should be consumed in moderation. While moderate caffeine consumption is generally seen as harmless, high consumption has been associated to fertility problems. Similarly, excessive alcohol use might upset hormonal equilibrium. Adopting attentive and moderate use of these substances is consistent with the larger goal of promoting reproductive health.

Fertility Foods to Avoid

Processed Foods: Inflammation Causing Agents

Reduce your intake of processed foods that are high in refined sugars, bad fats, and additives. These foods cause inflammation in the body, which can harm hormonal balance and reproductive health. To minimize inflammation, eat full, unprocessed foods.

Trans Fats Endangering Reproductive Health
Trans fats, which are found in partially hydrogenated oils and many processed snacks, should be avoided. Trans fats have been linked to an increased risk of infertility. To promote reproductive health, choose better fat sources such as olive oil, avocados, and almonds.

Excessive Caffeine Consumption: A Catch-22 Situation
While moderate caffeine consumption is generally seen as harmless, high consumption

has been associated to fertility problems. Caffeine use has been linked to delayed conception. Caffeine use should be reduced, especially if you intend to become pregnant.

High-Mercury Fish: A Word of Caution When Choosing Seafood

Excessive mercury exposure can affect reproductive health, therefore limit your diet of high-mercury fish. High-mercury fish include swordfish, shark, king mackerel, and tilefish. Choose low-mercury choices such as salmon and trout for omega-3 advantages without the hazards.

Excessive alcohol consumption disrupts hormonal balance.

Excessive alcohol use can alter hormonal balance and have an impact on fertility. While moderate alcohol use may have no effect, it is best to restrict alcohol consumption when actively attempting to conceive. Developing a mindful approach to alcohol is in line with the goal of improving reproductive health.

High Sugar Consumption Affects Insulin Sensitivity

Reduce your intake of meals and beverages high in added sugars. High sugar consumption can cause insulin resistance, disrupting hormonal balance and perhaps contributing to illnesses such as polycystic ovarian syndrome (PCOS). In moderation, choose whole foods and natural sweeteners.

Hormonal Regulation and Unhealthy Fats

Reduce your intake of harmful fats such as those found in fried foods, processed snacks, and some cooking oils. These fats can cause inflammation and interfere with hormone control. For better reproductive health, choose healthy fat sources including avocados, almonds, and olive oil.

Excessive Red Meat: How to Balance Protein Options

While lean foods are helpful, an overabundance of red and processed meats may be detrimental to fertility. Consumption of red meat has been linked to ovulatory infertility. Protein sources should be varied by including plant-based choices, fish, and lean poultry.

Unpasteurized Dairy and Cheese Pose an Infection Risk

Unpasteurized dairy products and soft cheeses manufactured from unpasteurized milk should be avoided. These items may pose a bacterial infection risk, which is especially concerning during pregnancy. To ensure safety, choose pasteurized dairy products.

Excess Soy: Balancing Phytoestrogen Intake

While soy can be part of a healthy diet, due to its phytoestrogen concentration, excessive consumption of soy-based products may disrupt hormonal balance. For individuals concerned about potential hormonal impacts, eating fermented soy products may be a better option.

Individualized Approaches and Expert Advice

Understanding that each person's physiology and lifestyle are distinct highlights the need of adapting dietary choices to specific demands. Seeking the advice of healthcare professionals, such as dietitians and fertility specialists, ensures a personalized strategy that takes into account issues such as preexisting health concerns, unique nutritional requirements, and lifestyle considerations. Individuals who receive personalized counsel are better able to make informed decisions that are in line with their reproductive goals as well as their overall well-being.

Making a Fertility-Inducing Plate

Navigating the fertility landscape with mindful dietary choices is a journey of empowerment and well-being. Individuals and couples can construct a fertility-boosting plate that coincides with the profound wisdom inscribed within the delicate dance of conception by eating a variety of nutrient-dense meals and avoiding those that may negatively impair reproductive health. Adopting this comprehensive approach to diet not only helps to optimize fertility, but it also builds a foundation for overall health and wellness.

CHAPTER 3

Lifestyle Factors

Stress Management's Influence on Fertility

The impact of stress in regulating fertility emerges as a significant factor amid the enthusiasm. Stress, a familiar companion in today's environment, can have far-reaching consequences for both physical and mental health. We delve into the delicate relationship between stress management and fertility in this comprehensive inquiry, seeking to understand how creating peace inside can pave the way for a more productive journey.

Untangling the Stress-Fertility Connection

Understanding Stress and the Body's Reaction

Stress is a normal and adaptive reaction to adversity, causing a cascade of physiological changes to prepare the body for a "fight or flight" scenario. While this response is necessary in an emergency, chronic stress - the continuous activation of the stress response - can be harmful to numerous biological systems.

Hormonal Balance in the Hypothalamus-Pituitary-Adrenal (HPA) Axis

The hypothalamic-pituitary-adrenal axis (HPA axis), a complex interplay between the hypothalamus, pituitary gland, and adrenal glands, is important to the body's stress response. When stressed, the hypothalamus produces corticotropin-releasing hormone (CRH), which signals the pituitary gland to produce adrenocorticotropic hormone (ACTH). As a result, the adrenal glands release cortisol, the primary stress hormone.

Reproductive Hormones and Chronic Stress

Chronic stress can disturb the delicate balance of reproductive hormones in the context of fertility. Elevated cortisol levels, a hallmark of chronic stress, may disrupt the normal functioning of the hypothalamus and pituitary gland, influencing the control of reproductive hormones like luteinizing hormone (LH) and follicle-stimulating hormone (FSH). These abnormalities can lead to irregular menstrual periods and ovulatory dysfunction in women, and sperm production and testosterone levels in males.

Stress and Fertility: A Mind-Body Connection

Conception Difficulties and Psychological Stress

The mind-body connection emphasizes the complex connections between psychological and physical health. Psychological stress can appear in physical symptoms and have an influence on fertility if it is caused by circumstances such as work pressure, marital troubles, or financial concerns. According to research, women with high levels of perceived stress may take longer to conceive than their less stressed counterparts.

Menstrual function and ovulation are affected.

Chronic stress can interfere with menstrual function and ovulation, making it difficult for women trying to conceive. Irregular menstrual periods and anovulation (lack of ovulation) are common symptoms of stress-induced reproductive system disturbances. Understanding these links emphasizes the necessity of managing stress as part of a comprehensive strategy to fertility.

The Effects of Stress on Male Fertility

Stress has an effect on male fertility as well. Chronic stress has been linked to changes in sperm characteristics such as concentration, motility, and shape. Stress can cause a drop in testosterone production and disturb the delicate process of sperm maturation. Recognizing the impact of stress in male fertility highlights the importance of a multifaceted approach that addresses the well-being of both couples.

Coping with Stress: Fertility Wellness Strategies

Developing Stress Management Techniques

Stress management is an important element of promoting reproductive wellness. Stress management methods can help individuals and couples on their fertility journey. Here are some methods to incorporate into your daily life:

Meditation for Mindfulness: Centering the Mind

The practice of mindfulness meditation entails paying attention to the current moment without judgment. Regular practice has been linked to lower stress levels and improved emotional well-being. Incorporating mindfulness into daily life, whether through guided meditation or mindful breathing exercises, is a useful approach for dealing with stress.

Yoga for Mind-Body Balance

Yoga blends physical postures, breathing exercises, and mindfulness to provide a comprehensive approach to stress treatment. Yoga practice not only improves flexibility and physical well-being, but it also improves mental clarity and emotional equilibrium. Yoga positions that target the pelvic area, for example, can be especially useful for conception.

Deep Breathing Techniques for Nervous System Calming

Deep breathing techniques, such as diaphragmatic or abdominal breathing, stimulate the relaxation response in the body. These strategies assist in the regulation of the autonomic nervous system, hence decreasing the impact of stress on the body. Deep breathing is a simple yet efficient approach to prevent the physiological impacts of stress.

Progressive Muscle Relaxation: Tension Release

Progressive muscle relaxation is tensing and then relaxing different muscle groups in order to promote physical and mental calm. Regular practice can help people become more in sync with their bodies and release tension that has built up during stressful times.

Emotional Support Through Counseling and Psychotherapy

Seeking counseling or psychotherapy can provide a secure space to explore and resolve underlying concerns. Professional assistance assists individuals in developing coping techniques, understanding stress triggers, and navigating the emotional difficulties connected with fertility challenges.

Art and Creativity: Creative Expression

Participating in artistic and creative endeavors provides a therapeutic outlet for expressing feelings and coping with stress. Individuals can channel their thoughts and experiences via painting, writing, or other kinds of creative expression, promoting a sense of empowerment and self-discovery.

Holistic Approaches to Fertility Wellness: Lifestyle Factors

Fertility and Physical Activity

Regular physical activity is essential for general health and can help with stress management and fertility. Exercise has been linked to mood improvements, stress reduction, and menstrual cycle control. However, balance is essential, as excessive exercise may have a negative impact on reproductive health. Finding a balanced strategy that meets individual tastes and needs promotes physical and emotional well-being.

Fertility and Nutrition

Nutrition is inextricably linked to fertility, and eating a well-balanced and healthy diet helps with general well-being. Choosing nutrient-dense foods, including a range of fruits and vegetables, and staying hydrated are all important components of a fertility-friendly diet. Furthermore, specific nutrients, such as omega-3 fatty acids and antioxidants, have been linked to improved reproductive health.

Restoring Vitality Through Sleep Hygiene

A good night's sleep is critical for general health and fertility. Sleep deprivation can contribute to increased stress, hormone abnormalities, and menstrual cycle irregularities. Consistent sleep habits, a pleasant sleeping environment, and emphasizing relaxation before bedtime all contribute to good sleep hygiene.

Building a Network for Social Support

The road to conception can be emotionally taxing, so having a supportive network is essential. Making relationships with friends, family, or support groups allows for the sharing of experiences, the exchange of viewpoints, and the promotion of emotional well-being. Social support protects against the effects of stress and fosters a sense of community.

Navigating the Fertility Landscape with Professional Assistance

Recognizing the complexities of reproductive issues, getting expert help is a proactive step toward full care. Fertility specialists, reproductive endocrinologists, and mental health practitioners who specialize in fertility concerns can offer tailored advice and support. Integrating medical and emotional treatment improves total fertility wellbeing.

Organizing Fertility Wellness

The congruence between stress management and reproductive wellbeing is obvious in the subtle dance of fertility. Individuals and couples can engage on a journey of deliberate well-being by understanding the physiological and psychological connection between stress and fertility. Stress management strategies, holistic lifestyle approaches, and seeking professional help all contribute to a symphony of wellness that echoes throughout the realms of mind and body. Let the music of self-care and harmony within lead us as we walk the paths to parenting, providing an atmosphere in which fertility can thrive.

Exercise and Fertility: The Road to Conception

Exercise appears as an important factor that not only helps to overall well-being but also connects with fertility. We dive into the complex relationship between exercise and conception in this exploration, revealing intricacies and providing insights for people and couples navigating the route to parenting.

The Relationship Between Exercise and Reproductive Health

Hormonal Balance and Physical Activity

Exercise has a significant impact on hormone regulation, which is important in reproductive health. Regular physical activity is linked to the release of endorphins, the body's natural mood elevators, which contribute to a feeling of well-being. Exercise also helps manage insulin levels, which can affect reproductive hormones including luteinizing hormone (LH) and follicle-stimulating hormone (FSH). It is critical for optimal fertility to achieve and maintain hormonal balance.

Fertility and Body Weight

The link between body weight and fertility is complex, and exercise is critical to maintaining a healthy weight. Excessive and insufficient body weight can both have an impact on reproductive function. Exercise can help obese people lose weight and improve their metabolic health, potentially increasing fertility. In contrast, for those who have lost weight owing to extreme exercise or restrictive food, regaining a healthy weight can improve reproductive hormone levels and monthly regularity.

Finding the Right Balance Between Exercise and Menstrual Regularity

Menstrual Cycle Effects

Menstrual regularity is an important predictor of reproductive health, and exercise can alter it in a variety of ways. Menstrual cycle disruptions may occur in some people, particularly those who participate in vigorous or excessive activity.

This condition, known as exercise-induced amenorrhea, is characterized by a lack of menstruation and is associated with hormonal abnormalities. Maintaining regular menstrual cycles and optimal fertility require a balance of exercise intensity and length.

The Female Athlete Triad Concept

The Female Athlete Triad refers to the conditions of disordered eating, amenorrhea, and osteoporosis, which are all linked. This triangle shows the potential repercussions of energy availability imbalances, which are common in female athletes undergoing intensive training. Managing and preventing the Female Athlete Triad requires addressing nutritional needs, moderating exercise intensity, and supporting hormonal balance.

Finding the Sweet Spot Between Exercise Intensity and Fertility

Fertility Advantages of Low-Intensity Exercise

Low-intensity exercise, such as brisk walking, swimming, or moderate yoga, has various reproductive benefits. These activities benefit overall cardiovascular health, stress management, and weight maintenance. Low-intensity exercise is generally well tolerated and is unlikely to impair reproductive function. Incorporating moderate-intensity activities into daily life can be a helpful start for persons wanting to maximize fertility.

Exercise at a Moderate Intensity: A Balanced Approach

Moderate-intensity exercise is a good middle ground between low and high-intensity activities. Activities in this category include jogging, cycling, and group fitness classes. Moderate exercise has been linked to gains in cardiovascular fitness, metabolic health, and mood. According to research, moderate-intensity exercise is unlikely to harm fertility and may even help to general reproductive well-being.

High-Intensity Exercise: Fertility Considerations

High-intensity exercise, defined by severe and demanding exercises, has piqued the interest of reproductive researchers. While research on the direct influence of high-intensity exercise on fertility is underway, some factors should be considered. Excessive activity, especially when combined with insufficient energy intake, might contribute to irregular menstrual cycles and hormonal disruptions. Striking a balance by adding rest and recovery intervals is critical for persons participating in high-intensity exercise while attempting to conceive.

Exercise Timing and Fertility: Insights for Conception

Preconception Exercise: Body Preparation
Regular exercise before attempting to conceive lays the groundwork for reproductive health. Preconception exercise improves general fitness, helps maintain a healthy body weight, and improves cardiovascular health. Establishing a routine that includes cardiovascular activities, strength training, and flexibility exercises lays the groundwork for a well-rounded approach to fitness that is compatible with fertility goals.

Exercise During the Menstrual Cycle

The menstrual cycle is separated into phases, each of which is marked by hormonal variations that can affect exercise tolerance and preferences. Understanding these periods might help you customize your workout regimen to best support your reproductive health.

Gentle Practices During Menstruation
Lower-intensity and mild exercises, such as strolling, yoga, or swimming, may be well-tolerated during the menstrual phase. These activities can aid with discomfort management and offer a supportive approach to self-care.

Follicular Phase: Endurance and Energy
Individuals' exercise tolerance frequently increases when their energy levels rise throughout the follicular phase. This phase is ideal for engaging in moderate-intensity

cardiovascular activities, strength training, and endurance and stamina-building activities.

Peak Performance During the Ovulatory Phase

The release of an egg during the ovulatory phase is related with enhanced energy and peak performance. If chosen, this phase allows individuals to engage in high-intensity activities. It is critical to listen to the body and select activities that correspond to individual preferences and comfort levels.

Mindful Movement During the Luteal Phase

Because of hormonal changes and possibly premenstrual symptoms, the luteal phase may necessitate more attentive and cautious activity. Yoga, Pilates, and other low-impact workouts can be beneficial at this stage.

A Holistic Approach to Nutrition, Hydration, and Exercise

Considerations for Active People's Nutrition

In the interaction between exercise and fertility, nutrition has a synergistic function. Active people should consume enough energy to sustain both their exercise performance and their reproductive health. Maintaining a well-balanced diet rich in nutrient-dense foods adds to general well-being.

Hydration is critical for both exercise and fertility.

Proper hydration is essential for people who exercise on a daily basis, and it also plays a role in fertility. Staying hydrated promotes overall biological functioning, such as the formation of cervical mucus, which helps sperm reach the egg. Maintaining proper water levels is critical for reproductive health.

Insights for Partners on Exercise and Male Fertility

Exercise has an impact on male reproductive health as well as fertility. Regular physical exercise has been linked to improved sperm parameters such as concentration, motility, and morphology. Excessive activity, on the other hand, especially when combined with factors such as heat exposure (e.g., frequent sauna use or tight-fitting sporting clothing), may have a deleterious impact on sperm quality. Striking a balance and exercising moderately are important considerations for male partners on the path to conception.

Individualized Guidance from Healthcare Professionals

While general guidelines can help, the relationship between exercise and fertility is highly individual. Consultation with healthcare professionals, such as fertility specialists and reproductive endocrinologists, provides tailored advice based on an individual's health status, reproductive objectives, and lifestyle considerations. Professional guidance can assist individuals in navigating fitness options, addressing specific difficulties, and developing a thorough strategy that corresponds with fertility goals.

Creating a Balanced Fertility and Fitness Approach

As individuals and couples embark on the path to motherhood, the link between exercise and fertility becomes clear. Developing a balanced strategy that takes into account exercise intensity, timing, and individual preferences benefits overall reproductive well-being. When handled attentively and in accordance with dietary and hydration requirements, exercise can be a beneficial ally on the road to conception. Individuals can empower themselves to navigate this difficult terrain by understanding the connection between physical exercise and fertility, encouraging a holistic approach that supports both health and the pursuit of a growing family.

CHAPTER 4

Environmental Influences

Uncovering the Health Effects of Toxins

Environmental variables play a key role in the intricate tapestry of factors impacting human health. Toxins in our environment, for example, pose challenges that affect many elements of our well-being. This investigation dives into the health impacts of pollutants, revealing the intricate linkages and throwing light on the significance of knowing and limiting their influence.

Toxins: A Multifaceted Environment

Pollutants in the Environment

Toxins are chemicals that can harm living beings. Toxins arise in a variety of forms and originate from a variety of sources in the context of environmental effects. Our exposure to these compounds is diverse, ranging from industrial pollutants and pesticides to naturally occurring poisons in certain plants and fungus. Understanding the many types of toxins and their routes into our life is critical for analyzing and managing their possible health implications.

Toxins Found in Everyday Life

Heavy Metals: Elements such as lead, mercury, and cadmium, which are frequently emitted by industrial activity, can contaminate the air, water, and soil. Chronic heavy metal exposure has been linked to negative effects on the brain system, kidneys, and other organs.

Pesticides and herbicides: These chemicals, which are used in agriculture to protect crops, may find their way into our food supply. Pesticide exposure has been related to a variety of health disorders, including reproductive issues and neurological impacts.

Air Quality: Particulate matter, volatile organic compounds (VOCs), and other air pollutants can be caused by vehicle emissions, industrial processes, and indoor activities. The health hazards connected with air pollution include respiratory disorders, cardiovascular problems, and systemic inflammation.

Endocrine Disruptors: Endocrine disruptors, which can be found in certain plastics, personal care products, and pesticides, interfere with the body's hormonal processes. This disturbance has been related to problems with reproduction, developmental defects, and an increased risk of some malignancies.

Toxin Effects on Health: Unraveling the Consequences

Effects on the Nervous System

Toxins, particularly heavy metals such as lead and mercury, have a significant impact on the neurological system. Lead exposure in children, whose developing brains are more vulnerable, can result in cognitive deficiencies, behavioral difficulties, and developmental delays. Mercury exposure is linked to neurological symptoms such as impaired memory, attention, and coordination.

Concerns about Reproductive Health

Toxins, particularly endocrine disruptors, can endanger reproductive health. These chemicals may disrupt hormonal signaling, resulting in menstruation abnormalities, decreased fertility, and pregnancy difficulties. Toxin exposure during pregnancy has been associated with developmental problems in offspring.

Respiratory Problems

Particulate matter and VOCs, for example, are airborne contaminants that can harm respiratory health. Long-term exposure has been linked to asthma, chronic obstructive pulmonary disease (COPD), and an increased risk of respiratory infections. Children's respiratory systems are still developing, making them especially vulnerable.

Effects on the Cardiovascular System

Environmental pollutants have an influence on the cardiovascular system. For example, air pollution has been related to an increased risk of cardiovascular disorders such as heart attacks and strokes. Pollutants inhaled can cause inflammation and oxidative stress, which can contribute to the development and progression of cardiovascular disease.

Cancer Dangers

Certain poisons are classified as carcinogens, which means they have the potential to cause cancer. Prolonged exposure to chemicals such as asbestos, benzene, and some pesticides has been linked to an increased chance of developing cancer. Understanding and avoiding recognized carcinogens are critical measures in cancer prevention.

Strategies for a Healthier Environment: Mitigating Exposure

Environmental Education and Advocacy

Raising awareness about environmental toxins and campaigning for regulations that limit their use and emissions are critical steps toward a healthier environment. Individuals contribute to the collective effort to protect public health by supporting measures that limit the discharge of poisons into the air, water, and soil.

Consumer Preferences and Environmentally Friendly Practices

Making informed purchase choices is critical to lowering human exposure to pollutants. Choosing organic produce, household products with few chemical ingredients, and eco-friendly alternatives all contribute to a better living environment. Adopting sustainable behaviors, such as eliminating single-use plastics and supporting environmentally conscious businesses, is in line with attempts to reduce the overall impact of toxins.

Improving Air Quality

Given the serious health dangers posed by air pollution, efforts to enhance air quality are critical. This involves campaigning for cleaner energy sources, supporting public transit programs, and putting in place industrial emission-reduction measures. Individuals can also help by lowering their personal contributions to air pollution, such as driving less and using energy-efficient equipment.

Toxin Analysis and Monitoring

Environmental toxin levels are regularly tested

and monitored, providing vital data for assessing potential dangers and executing targeted treatments. This includes monitoring the quality of the air and water, particularly in areas with industrial activity or a history of toxin contamination. Proactive monitoring allows for quick reactions to developing environmental risks.

Towards a Healthier Tomorrow

Recognizing the impact of toxins on health is a critical step toward fostering collective well-being as we traverse the complex landscape of environmental influences. Environmental poisons have far-reaching consequences, ranging from neurological impairments to reproductive health difficulties. We may aim for a healthier tomorrow through a combination of awareness, advocacy, and individual choices—one in which the air we breathe, the water we drink, and the spaces we inhabit contribute to the vitality and resilience of both current and future generations. Each step taken toward reducing toxic exposure is a step closer to a future where health and environmental harmony coexist.

Making Your Environment Fertility-Friendly

Environmental influences can affect fertility in a variety of ways, ranging from minor changes in hormone balance to more dramatic effects on reproductive organs. Chemical contaminants, lifestyle decisions, and even the quality of air and water can all contribute to an individual's or couple's overall reproductive health. Recognizing the potential impact of the environment on fertility emphasizes the need of creating environments that promote conception.

Environmental Factors Influencing Fertility

Endocrine Disruptors: Endocrine disruptors, which can be found in certain plastics, personal care products, and pesticides, can disturb hormonal equilibrium. This disruption may contribute to menstruation abnormalities, decreased fertility, and pregnancy problems.

Pollutants in the air, such as particulate matter and volatile organic compounds (VOCs), have been linked to respiratory problems and an increased chance of miscarriage. Because people spend so much of their time indoors, maintaining appropriate indoor air quality is very important.

Chemical Exposures: Certain chemicals, whether in the workplace or in everyday life, can have an affect on fertility. Workplace exposure to solvents and industrial chemicals, for example, may endanger reproductive health.

Smoking, excessive alcohol intake, and a sedentary lifestylc can all have an impact on fertility. Addressing these lifestyle factors to enhance general well-being is part of creating a fertility-friendly environment.

Practical Strategies for Creating a Fertility-Friendly Home

Conscious Purchases of Household Goods

Choose Natural Cleaning Products:

Choose cleaning products that do not include harsh chemicals or poisons. Natural alternatives, such as vinegar, baking soda, and lemon, can clean well while exposing you to less toxic elements. Many environmentally friendly cleaning companies provide products that promote both cleanliness and environmental safety.

Think about organic bedding and mattresses:

Organic bedding and mattresses decrease exposure to harmful chemicals contained in conventional bedding. Choose organic cotton sheets and mattresses that do not include flame retardants or other chemicals.

Personal Care Product Evaluation:

Examine personal care goods, such as lotions, shampoos, and cosmetics, for potentially dangerous components. Look for products with less chemical additives, and consider buying organic or natural products. This includes both partners' items.

Maintaining Indoor Air Quality

Ventilate Living Rooms:

Maintaining healthy indoor air quality requires proper ventilation. Open windows on a regular basis to allow fresh air to flow, and think about utilizing air purifiers with HEPA filters to decrease airborne pollutants.

Mindful Paint Selections:

Choose paints with minimal or no volatile organic compounds (VOCs) when redecorating or renovating. VOCs can emit toxic substances into the atmosphere, affecting indoor air quality.

Reduce your exposure to tobacco smoke:

If possible, try to make your workplace smoke-free. Both active smoking and secondhand smoke exposure have been linked to reproductive difficulties and pregnancy concerns.

Nutrition and Lifestyle Choices

Adopt a Well-Balanced Diet: Nutrition is critical to reproductive health. Choose a diet high in fruits, vegetables, whole grains, lean proteins, and healthy fats. Consume enough important nutrients, such as folate, iron, and omega-3 fatty acids.

Keep Hydrated: Hydration is critical to general health, especially reproductive health. Drinking enough water promotes optimal biological functioning, such as the formation of cervical mucus, which aids sperm in reaching the egg.

Moderate Exercise Program: Regular moderate-intensity exercise can help you feel better overall. Physical activity helps with hormone balance, stress management, and cardiovascular health, all of which are favorable to conception.

Making a Relaxing Sleep Environment

Make sleep hygiene a priority:

Maintain a consistent sleep schedule, create a comfortable sleep environment, and practice relaxation techniques before bedtime to develop healthy sleep habits. Sleep is critical for reproductive health.

Purchase a Comfortable Mattress:

A sturdy and comfortable mattress might help you sleep better. Choose a mattress that fits your needs and provides adequate spinal support.

Stress Management:

In order to produce a tranquil and relaxed sleeping environment, incorporate stress management strategies into your daily life. Before bedtime, this could include mindfulness meditation, deep breathing exercises, or gentle stretching.

Nature Connection and Outdoor Spaces

Develop Green Spaces:

Greenery should be included into living spaces wherever possible. Indoor plants not only improve air quality by filtering out harmful toxins, but they also offer aesthetic value.

Spend Time Outside:

Spending time outside on a regular basis, whether in parks, gardens, or natural settings, allows you to connect with nature. Nature exposure has been linked to stress reduction and overall well-being.

Sun Exposure with Caution:

Sun exposure should be balanced with sun safety to ensure optimal vitamin D production. Vitamin D is necessary for reproductive health, and moderate sun exposure can help the body synthesize it.

Seeking Professional Help

While developing a fertility-friendly atmosphere necessitates deliberate choices and behaviors, it is critical to remember that individual circumstances differ. Seeking advice from healthcare professionals, such as fertility specialists and reproductive endocrinologists, ensures a customized approach that takes into account unique health issues, reproductive goals, and probable challenges.

Growing Fertility in Every Corner

The environment in which individuals and couples live plays an important part in the intricate fabric of fertility. Individuals can help to optimize reproductive wellbeing by mindfully creating a fertility-friendly refuge. From making mindful choices in household products to improving indoor air quality and embracing fertility-friendly lifestyle behaviors, each step contributes to the overall well-being of both partners. Let every area of our living spaces vibrate with the harmony of fertility as we walk the route to motherhood, nourishing the seeds of life with a setting that speaks to the profound connection between health, wellbeing, and the promise of new beginnings.

CHAPTER 5

Nourishing the Journey

The Importance of Nutrients

Essential nutrients occupy center stage in the arena of nutrition, playing a critical role in sustaining body processes and boosting general well-being. This investigation dives into the importance of key nutrients, focusing light on their various roles and emphasizing their critical contribution to the nourishing journey.

The Vitality of Essential Nutrients

Identifying and Classifying Essential Nutrients

The term "essential nutrients" refers to substances that the body requires for proper functioning but cannot create in sufficient quantities, necessitating their intake through the diet. These nutrients are required for a variety of physiological functions, ranging from energy metabolism to the maintenance of structural integrity in tissues.

Essential Nutrient Categories

Vitamins:

Vitamins are organic chemicals that are essential in a variety of biological activities. Each vitamin has distinct roles that are important for overall well-being, ranging from supporting immune function (vitamin C) to boosting bone health (vitamin D).

Minerals:

Minerals are inorganic elements that are required for a wide range of physiological functions. Calcium, for example, is essential for bone health, but iron is essential for oxygen transport through the blood.

Proteins:

Proteins are amino acid-based molecules that are essential for the structure, function, and control of the body's tissues and organs. Because the body cannot generate essential amino acids on its own, they must be received from diet.

Essential Fatty Acids (Fats):

Essential fatty acids, such as omega-3 and omega-6, are essential for cellular structure and function. They are essential for brain health, cardiovascular function, and inflammatory reactions.

Carbohydrates:

While carbs are not usually considered vital, they are the body's principal source of energy.

Choosing complex carbs, such as whole grains and veggies, gives long-lasting energy as well as critical elements.

Essential Nutrients' Multifaceted Roles

Macronutrients and Energy Metabolism

Carbohydrates:

Carbohydrates are the body's principal energy source. They are converted into glucose, which powers cellular functions. Choosing complex carbs ensures a continuous flow of energy, which aids in the maintenance of bodily processes.

Proteins:

Proteins are important in energy metabolism because they provide energy when carbs are lacking. Proteins are also required for the creation of enzymes, hormones, and structural components such as muscles and connective tissues.

Fats:

Essential fatty acids aid in energy metabolism and the absorption of fat-soluble vitamins (A, D, E, and K). They are an essential component of cell membrane structure, supporting cellular function and integrity.

Micronutrients and Structure Support

Calcium:

Calcium is required for the development and maintenance of strong bones and teeth. It is also essential for muscular contraction, blood clotting, and nerve transmission.

Iron:

Iron is an essential component of hemoglobin, the molecule that transports oxygen in the blood. Adequate iron consumption is critical for avoiding anemia and maintaining general health.

Vitamins:

Vitamins help with a variety of structural and regulatory roles. Vitamin C, for example, is required for collagen formation, which supports skin, cartilage, and blood vessels. Vitamin A aids in the maintenance of good vision.

Antioxidant Defense and Immune Function

Vitamins C and E:

These vitamins function as antioxidants, removing free radicals that can harm cells. They are essential for immunological function and safeguarding the organism from oxidative damage.

Selenium and zinc:

Minerals such as zinc and selenium help to maintain immunological health. Zinc aids immune cell activity, whereas selenium aids in the creation of antioxidant enzymes.

Brain Health and Cognitive Function

Fatty Acids Omega-3:

Omega-3 fatty acids, in particular, are critical for brain health and cognitive function. They help to support neurotransmitter activity by contributing to the construction of cell membranes in the brain.

Vitamin B:

B vitamins, such as B6, B9 (folate), and B12, are important for brain function. They play a role in neurotransmitter synthesis and the upkeep of the myelin sheath, a protective covering of nerve fibers.

Using Supplements to Fill Nutritional Gaps

Choosing Supplements Wisely

While a well-balanced diet should ideally contain all important elements, certain circumstances may result in nutritional deficiencies. Dietary restrictions, special health issues, or lifestyle choices may need the use of supplements to maintain adequate nutritional intake.

Vitamin D:

Vitamin D, which is necessary for calcium absorption and bone health, is generated in the skin when exposed to sunshine. Individuals with limited sun exposure or specific medical issues, on the other hand, may benefit from vitamin D pills.

Fatty Acids Omega-3:
Getting enough omega-3 fatty acids, which are found in fatty fish, flaxseeds, and walnuts, is essential for cardiovascular and neurological health. Omega-3 supplements, such as fish oil, are a practical option for people who don't get enough omega-3s from their diet.

Iron:
Iron deficiency is a widespread worry, especially for people who follow strict diets or have high iron requirements. Iron supplements may be

prescribed for persons at risk of insufficiency, but professional assistance is required to avoid excessive ingestion.

Folate:

Folate, a B vitamin, is required during pregnancy for cell division and the prevention of neural tube abnormalities. Folate supplements are frequently suggested for pregnant women or those planning to get pregnant.

The Art of Nutritional Harmony: A Balancing Act

Synergy of Nutrients and Whole Foods

Consume a Rainbow:

Consuming a variety of fruits and vegetables provides a wide range of vitamins, minerals, and antioxidants. Different hues frequently represent diverse nutrient profiles, which contributes to total nutritional diversity.

Combining Nutrient-Dense Foods:

Increase vitamin absorption by strategically combining foods. Consuming vitamin C-rich foods alongside iron-containing plant sources, for example, enhances iron absorption. Nutrient synergy throughout entire foods boosts their overall impact.

Individualized Nutritional Approaches

Consider Specific Requirements:

Individual nutrient requirements are influenced by factors such as age, gender, life stage, and unique health issues. Personalizing food choices and, when appropriate, supplement regimens to fulfill these specific needs promotes personalized nutritional well-being.

Professional Advice:

Consultation with healthcare professionals, such as qualified dietitians and nutritionists, provides tailored advice. These experts can assess individual nutrient requirements, address dietary problems, and provide evidence-based recommendations.

Developing Nutritional Resilience

Essential nutrients emerge as the choreographers in the intricate dance of health and wellness, directing the symphony of body activities and supporting the journey to optimal well-being. Essential nutrients are the foundations of feeding, from their fundamental roles in energy metabolism to their intricate contributions to structural integrity. Individuals who embrace the art of balance, variety, and mindfulness as they walk the pathways of nutrition build a canvas of nutritional resilience. Essential nutrients are the building blocks that pave the way for a life rich in vigor, resilience, and the long-term pursuit of health, whether taken from vibrant whole foods or supplemented with care.

Supplements Suggestions

While nutrition and lifestyle decisions are the foundation of fertility, certain circumstances may need the strategic use of supplements to improve chances of conception. This comprehensive guide navigates the landscape of fertility-specific supplements, providing insights into their roles, potential advantages, and considerations for people on the route to creating new life.

Nutrient Balance Is Critical:

Fertility is inextricably linked to general health, and a well-balanced diet provides the cornerstone for reproductive well-being. Essential nutrients are important for hormonal balance, egg and sperm production, and general reproductive health.

Taking Care of Nutrient Deficiencies:

Nutrient shortages can have an impact on fertility. It is critical for both couples to maintain adequate amounts of important vitamins and minerals, as deficits can interfere with the delicate processes of conception and early pregnancy.

Fertility Supplements to Consider

Folate:

Folate is a B-vitamin that is essential for reproductive health. It assists in the production of DNA and has been linked to a lower risk of neural tube abnormalities. Both spouses should get enough folate, either through food or supplementation.

Iron:

Iron is essential for both male and female reproduction. Maintaining adequate iron levels in women promotes overall health and lowers the risk of anemia, which can disrupt menstrual periods. Men who are iron deficient may have poor sperm quality.

Vitamin D:

Vitamin D is necessary for hormonal balance and may improve conception. It helps women's menstrual cycles and men's testosterone levels. Adequate vitamin D levels can be achieved with adequate sunshine exposure and supplementation.

Fatty Acids Omega-3:

Omega-3 fatty acids, specifically DHA and EPA, are favorable to reproductive health. They help to maintain hormonal balance, improve egg and sperm quality, and may increase the likelihood of successful fertility treatments.

CoQ10 (Coenzyme Q10):

CoQ10 is an antioxidant that aids in the creation of energy within cells. It has been linked to better egg and sperm quality, making it an important supplement for couples trying to conceive.

Zinc:

Zinc is essential for both male and female fertility. It helps to produce healthy eggs and sperm, and deficits can cause hormonal abnormalities. Zinc supplements may be advantageous for people who do not get enough zinc from their diet.

Vitamin E:

Vitamin E is an antioxidant that may help with conception. It protects cells from oxidative stress and promotes male and female reproductive health. Including vitamin E-rich foods and supplements in your diet can help with fertility.

L-arginine:

L-arginine is an amino acid that promotes blood flow to reproductive organs by acting as a vasodilator. This is especially useful for men, as increased blood flow to the genitals may boost sperm quality.

Choosing Supplements Wisely for Fertility Goals

Preconception Preparation

Multivitamins for Preconception:
Preconception multivitamins for both couples can provide a full array of important nutrients. In suitable quantities, these formulations frequently include fertility-supporting vitamins and minerals.

Individualized Requirements:
When choosing supplements, keep in mind your personal reproductive requirements. Age, previous health issues, and individual fertility challenges may all influence the supplements chosen for maximum support.

Supplements for Male Fertility

Selenium:

Selenium is a trace element that has been linked to male fertility. It is involved in the formation and function of sperm. Consuming selenium-rich meals and supplements may help increase sperm quality.

Men's Folic Acid:

While folic acid is generally connected with female fertility, it is equally important for men. It promotes the health of sperm and the integrity of DNA. In addition to food sources, men should consider folic acid supplements.

Fertility Support and Lifestyle Factors

Supplements High in Antioxidants:

Antioxidants including vitamin C, vitamin E, and selenium aid in the neutralization of oxidative stress, which can impair fertility.

Selecting antioxidant-rich supplements may benefit both partners.

Supplements for the mind-body connection:
Stress reduction is essential for fertility. Magnesium and B-vitamin supplements can help the neurological system and contribute to overall well-being, which can improve fertility outcomes.

Consultation with Fertility Experts

Individualized Fertility Strategies

Professional Advice:
Consultation with fertility specialists, such as reproductive endocrinologists and fertility-focused healthcare providers, enables tailored examinations and suggestions. These

experts can create supplement regimens to address specific reproductive issues.

Fertility Evaluation:

Undergoing relevant testing before and throughout fertility-focused supplementation can provide insights into hormone levels, nutritional status, and potential areas of concern. This data informs the establishment of a targeted fertility plan.

Supplementation Monitoring and Adjustment

Regular Evaluations:

It is critical to regularly assess fertility and change supplement regimens as needed. Fertility specialists can perform assessments and make recommendations to improve the odds of conception.

Addressing the Root Causes:

Fertility-focused healthcare providers can diagnose and treat underlying fertility difficulties. This could include a combination of lifestyle changes, medical procedures, and supplement recommendations.

Fertility Support Through Informed Supplementation

As couples embark on the complicated journey of fertility, the function of prescribed supplements in maintaining reproductive health becomes a focus point. Strategic supplementation helps to create new life by treating dietary deficits and improving the quality of eggs and sperm.

Each nutrient serves a distinct part in the tapestry of fertility, contributing to the complicated dance of conception. Individuals and couples can traverse this journey with confidence and resilience by making informed choices, following individualized supplementation strategies, and seeking the advice of reproductive professionals. May the road to motherhood be distinguished not only by a strong yearning for new beginnings, but also by the deliberate and nurturing support of fertility through the strategic inclusion of prescribed supplements.

Supplement Side Effects and Suitability How Fertility Supplements Work

Fertility supplements frequently include a blend of vitamins, minerals, antioxidants, and herbal extracts. These components are intended to address nutritional deficiencies, promote reproductive organ health, and increase overall fertility. Common ingredients include folic acid, zinc, coenzyme Q10, and numerous plant extracts purported to boost fertility.

Side Effects of Fertility Supplements

While fertility drugs are generally seen to be safe, it is vital to be aware of any possible side effects. These can vary depending on the individual's health and the specific substances in the supplement. Common side effects include stomach upset, allergic reactions to certain herbs, and drug interactions.

1. Digestive Discomfort: Some patients may experience digestive discomfort, such as nausea, bloating, or stomach pain. This is commonly associated with specific substances, and adjusting the dosage or taking the supplement with food may be beneficial.

2. Allergy Reactions: Some people are allergic to botanical extracts contained in fertility supplements. Before using supplements, be aware of any known allergies to the ingredients and consult with a medical professional.

3. Drug Interactions: Fertility supplements and medications can interact, potentially lowering efficacy or causing adverse reactions. Individuals who are using medications for pre-existing conditions should consult their doctor before beginning fertility supplements.

4. Excessive vitamin and mineral consumption:

Excessive use of some vitamins and minerals, such as vitamin A, vitamin D, or iron, may be harmful. It is crucial to follow the dosage instructions and avoid taking additional supplements, which could result in an accidental overdose.

Who Can Benefit From Fertility Supplements?

1. persons with Nutritional Deficiencies: Fertility supplements may be beneficial to persons who have nutritional deficiencies. Low folic acid or zinc levels, for example, may have an effect on fertility, and supplements can help correct these deficiencies.

2. Couples Going Through Fertility Treatments: Fertility supplements may benefit those going through fertility treatments including in vitro fertilization (IVF). These therapies can be physically taxing, and vitamins may be beneficial to general health.

3. Pregnant Women: Women who are trying to conceive may want to explore fertility pills as a precautionary measure. Maintaining proper nutritional levels prior to conception can boost fertility and help to a healthy pregnancy.

Who Should Avoid Fertility Supplements?

1. People with Pre-existing Medical Condition: Individuals with pre-existing medical conditions, such as diabetes, cardiovascular disease, or autoimmune disorders, should exercise extreme caution while contemplating fertility supplements. Certain components may interact with medications or exacerbate pre-existing medical issues.

2. People on Multiple Medications: Those on multiple medications should consult their doctor before commencing fertility supplements. Interactions have the potential to impair medicinal efficacy or create undesired side effects.

3. Allergy Proneness: People who are allergic or sensitive to herbal extracts should exercise extreme caution. Allergic reactions to certain components can range from mild to severe, thus it is vital to be fully aware of potential allergens.

4. Women who are pregnant or breastfeeding:
Pregnant or lactating women should take caution when taking fertility tablets. Certain substances may be harmful to ingest while pregnant, thus it is vital to consult with a healthcare professional to ensure the safety of both the individual and the developing fetus.

Making Informed Decisions Is Critical
Including fertility supplements in one's reproductive health routine requires careful consideration and decision-making. Before embarking on any supplement regimen, individuals and couples should perform the following:

1. Seek Advice from Medical Professionals: It is vital to seek advice from medical professionals such as gynecologists or fertility specialists. These professionals can assess a person's health, detect potential hazards, and provide specific recommendations.

2. Submit to Preconception Testing: Preconception testing can help detect specific nutritional deficiencies or health issues that may impair fertility. This information guides personalized supplementing based on individual needs.

3. Extensive Ingredient Research: Understanding the ingredients in fertility pills is crucial. Thorough research, including potential side effects and interactions, enables consumers to make informed health-related decisions.

4. Monitor for Changes: It is vital to regularly assess how the body reacts to supplements.

Individuals should immediately contact their healthcare providers if they have any adverse reactions or unexpected changes so that the regimen can be changed as needed.

Fertility supplements can be valuable in the pursuit of reproductive health, but they must be used in conjunction with a well-balanced and knowledgeable strategy. Recognizing potential side effects, comprehending individual suitability, and collaborating with healthcare specialists all contribute to a well-rounded fertility wellness strategy.

In the complicated landscape of reproductive health, each person's journey is unique. Individuals and couples can proceed with confidence if they navigate fertility supplements with knowledge and caution, knowing that their selections are based on understanding and a commitment to total well-being.

CHAPTER 6

Understanding Male Fertility

Examining Male Factors

While conversations frequently focus on women's health and fertility, understanding male characteristics is equally important. This in-depth investigation dives into the diverse world of male fertility, elucidating the biological, lifestyle, and environmental aspects that influence reproductive health.

The Basis of Male Fertility

Biological Fundamentals

Spermatogenesis:

The process of spermatogenesis—the ongoing generation of sperm cells in the testes—is the foundation of male fertility. The development of germ cells into functional sperm, ready to embark on the journey toward fertilization, is a complex biochemical dance.

Hormonal Balance:

Hormones conduct the male reproductive function symphony. The pituitary gland secretes follicle-stimulating hormone (FSH) and luteinizing hormone (LH), which increase testosterone production and sperm generation in the testes. This precise hormonal balance is required for proper fertility.

Recognizing Male Reproductive Anatomy

Terrain Testicular

Sperm and Testes Production:

The testes, located in the scrotum, contain seminiferous tubules that produce sperm. Sperm then passes through the epididymis, maturing and becoming motile—a critical stage in the process of fertilization.

Production of sperm:

Aside from sperm, the seminal vesicles, prostate, and bulbourethral glands all contribute to the production of sperm. During ejaculation, this seminal fluid nourishes and transports sperm, increasing their chances of reaching the egg.

Male Fertility Influencing Factors

Contributors from the biological realm

Genetic Variables:

Male fertility can be affected by genetic abnormalities. Klinefelter syndrome, Y chromosome deletions, and chromosomal abnormalities can all have an impact on sperm production, motility, and morphology.

Varicocele:

A varicocele is an expansion of veins in the scrotum that can lead to testicular hyperthermia. This higher temperature may impair sperm production and quality, reducing fertility overall.

Hormonal Balance

Levels of Testosterone:

The principal male sex hormone, testosterone, is critical for sperm production and overall reproductive health. Imbalances in testosterone levels may have an impact on fertility, highlighting the interconnection of hormonal control.

Levels of FSH and LH:

Follicle-stimulating hormone (FSH) and luteinizing hormone (LH) are important regulators of spermatogenesis. Changes in their levels can have an effect on sperm production and maturation, influencing male fertility.

Male Fertility and Lifestyle Factors

Food and Nutrition

Diet High in Antioxidants:

Antioxidants, which are present in fruits, vegetables, and nuts, protect against oxidative stress. Including antioxidant-rich foods in one's diet may improve sperm quality and minimize DNA damage.

Consumption of zinc and folate:

Zinc and folate levels must be adequate for sperm formation and function. Zinc promotes sperm motility, while folate helps to maintain the integrity of sperm DNA.

Physical Activity and Body Weight

Obesity's Effect:

Obesity is linked to hormonal abnormalities, specifically higher estrogen levels. This can have a negative impact on sperm production and quality. Maintaining a healthy weight is critical for fertility.

Moderation in Exercise:

While regular exercise is good for your overall health, excessive and severe physical activity can have an influence on your fertility. It is critical to strike a balance that promotes cardiovascular health while minimizing stress on the reproductive system.

Environmental Risks

Chemical Contamination:

Environmental contaminants such as pesticides, industrial chemicals, and heavy metals can have an effect on male fertility. Reduced exposure and preventative actions contribute to reproductive health.

Heat Exposed:

Prolonged exposure to high temperatures, such as hot baths, saunas, or wearing tight underwear, might raise testicular temperature and potentially affect sperm production. Being aware of heat exposure promotes good fertility.

Tobacco, Alcohol, and Substance Abuse

The Effects of Smoking:

Cigarette smoking has been associated with decreased sperm count, motility, and morphology. Tobacco use causes DNA damage in sperm, stressing the necessity of quitting smoking for fertility.

The Effects of Alcohol:

Excessive alcohol consumption can disturb hormonal balance and have a negative impact on sperm quality. Alcohol consumption in moderation or abstinence contributes to a healthy reproductive environment.

Use of Substances:

Illicit substance usage, such as marijuana and cocaine, has been linked to male fertility problems. Substance misuse can impair hormonal control, affecting sperm production and function directly.

Psychosocial Factors Influencing Male Fertility

Stress and Mental Health

Stress Effect:

Chronic stress can cause hormonal abnormalities and interfere with sperm development. Stress management approaches, such as meditation and relaxation exercises, benefit both mental health and fertility.

Psychological Aspects:

Anxiety and sadness, for example, can have an effect on sexual function and libido. Addressing mental health issues through therapy or counseling improves overall reproductive health.

Male Fertility and Medical Conditions

Chronic Diseases

Diabetes Relationship:

Diabetes, particularly uncontrolled diabetes, can have an impact on male fertility. Elevated blood sugar levels can cause oxidative stress and damage to sperm, emphasizing the necessity of diabetes management for reproductive health.

Cardiovascular Disease and Hypertension:

Blood flow, particularly circulation to the vaginal area, can be affected by hypertension and cardiovascular disorders. Maintaining cardiovascular health is essential for reproductive function.

Male Fertility and Age

Changes with Age:

Male fertility can diminish with age, though not as sharply as in women. Advanced paternal age has been linked to a steady decline in sperm quality and an increased chance of child genetic disorders.

Fertility Testing and Professional Advice

Examination of sperm

Parameters of sperm:

Semen analysis evaluates important factors such as sperm count, motility, and morphology. Understanding these parameters provides vital insights into male reproductive health and serves as a direction for future research.

When to Look for Testing:

Couples who are having trouble conceiving might seek fertility testing. If conception does not occur after a year of regular, unprotected intercourse, professional help is recommended.

Consultation with Fertility Experts

Andrologists' Role:

Andrologists, or male reproductive health professionals, are critical in identifying and resolving male fertility concerns. Consulting with andrologists ensures a thorough evaluation and individualized treatment strategy.

Approach Based on Collaboration:

Fertility testing is frequently a collaborative effort involving both couples. Collaboration with reproductive endocrinologists and fertility specialists can assist you manage the complexities of fertility issues.

Male Fertility Treatment Alternatives

Interventions in Medicine

Hormonal Treatments:

Hormonal imbalances that affect fertility can be treated with hormonal treatments. These treatments are intended to restore hormonal balance and promote healthy sperm production.

Surgical Procedures:

Varicoceles or blockages in the reproductive tract may necessitate surgical surgery. These operations are designed to address anatomical abnormalities that are impeding sperm production or transmission.

Changes in Lifestyle

Dietary Modifications:
Adopting a fertility-friendly diet high in antioxidants, zinc, and folate improves reproductive health overall. Dietary changes help to create a nutrient-rich environment for sperm production.

Weight Control:
Having and maintaining a healthy weight has a positive impact on hormonal balance and sperm quality. To address obesity-related reproductive

difficulties, weight management techniques may be prescribed.

Psychosocial Assistance

Services for Counseling and Support:
Psychological assistance is essential during the conception process. Throughout the process, counseling services give individuals and couples coping techniques, stress management tactics, and emotional support.

Educational Materials:
Access to educational resources and support groups raises awareness and comprehension of male fertility issues. Peer support and shared experiences help to build community and resilience.

Navigating the Male Fertility Tapestry

Male factors weave a vital thread in the delicate tapestry of fertility, affecting the landscape of reproductive health for couples globally. Understanding the biological complexities, recognizing the impact of lifestyle choices, and recognizing the influence of psychological factors are all important stages in navigating the complexities of male fertility.

As individuals and couples embark on the path to fatherhood, the collective wisdom gained by peeling back the layers of male fertility aids in making educated decisions. The route forward is paved with knowledge, perseverance, and the shared desire to nurture the gift of new life, from adopting a holistic approach to fertility to seeking professional support when necessary. May this thorough investigation serve as a compass, guiding those on the path to motherhood through the thorny terrain of male fertility with understanding, compassion, and everlasting optimism.

Methods for Improving Sperm Quality

The quality of sperm is critical in the road to conception in the complicated dance of fertility. Understanding the factors that influence sperm quality and implementing techniques to maximize reproductive potential are critical for couples hoping to start a family. This comprehensive book delves into a variety of techniques to improving sperm quality, covering biological, lifestyle, and environmental issues that all contribute to the delicate balance of male reproductive health.

Uncovering the Sperm Quality Dynamics

Sperm Function and Composition

The Importance of Sperm Quality

Sperm quality includes several factors such as sperm count, motility, and morphology. These elements jointly impact sperm's reproductive potential and capacity to effectively fertilize an egg.

Integrity of DNA:

The integrity of sperm DNA is an important factor in sperm quality. Damage to sperm DNA can impair fertility, causing difficulties in conception and perhaps having an impact on offspring's health.

Sperm Quality Influenced by Biological Factors

Hormonal and Genetic Dynamics

Genetic Factors:

Genetic variables can have an effect on sperm production and function. Understanding one's genetic profile and resolving any abnormalities that are discovered are critical for maximizing sperm quality.

Hormonal Harmony:

Hormonal balance, particularly with regard to testosterone, FSH, and LH, is critical for spermatogenesis. Imbalances can have a negative impact on sperm production and quality, highlighting the importance of hormonal health.

Lifestyle Changes to Improve Sperm Quality

Food and Nutrition

Diet High in Antioxidants:

Antioxidants protect sperm from oxidative stress, which can harm it. Consuming fruits, vegetables, nuts, and whole grains gives a good amount of antioxidants.

Supplementation with zinc:

Zinc is essential for the generation and quality of sperm. Consider including zinc-rich meals or supplements to help maintain appropriate levels for better reproductive health.

Fatty Acids Omega-3

Important Fats for Sperm Health:

Omega-3 fatty acids, which can be found in fish, flaxseeds, and walnuts, help to maintain sperm membrane integrity and motility. Including these vital lipids in your diet improves sperm quality overall.

Supplements made from fish oil:
Supplements can provide a concentrated amount of omega-3 fatty acids for those with a low dietary consumption, promoting the absorption of these important lipids into sperm cell membranes.

Folate Supports DNA Integrity

Foods High in Folate:
Folate is required for the production and repair of DNA. Consuming folate-rich foods such as leafy greens, legumes, and fortified cereals helps to maintain sperm DNA integrity.

Folic acid supplementation:

Folic acid supplementation is recommended, especially for people who do not get enough folate from their diet. This can help to keep sperm health at an optimal level.

Changes in Lifestyle to Improve Sperm Quality

Weight Control

Obesity's Impact:
Obesity is associated with hormonal abnormalities and might have a negative impact on sperm quality. Adopting a good weight-management plan benefits reproductive health.

Exercise on a regular basis:
Regular moderate-intensity exercise benefits overall health, including reproductive health.

Physical activity helps to maintain hormonal balance and sperm production.

Temperature Control

Preventing Overheating:

Prolonged exposure to high temperatures, such as hot baths or wearing tight underwear, might raise testicular temperature and affect sperm production. Avoiding warming promotes sperm quality.

Showers that are too cold:

Cold showers or brief exposure to cold temperatures can aid with testicular temperature regulation. This simple exercise helps to create an atmosphere conducive to sperm production.

Lowering Stress Levels

Sperm Quality and Stress:

Chronic stress may have an adverse effect on sperm production and function. Stress management approaches, such as mindfulness or meditation, benefit both mental and reproductive health.

Relaxation should be prioritized:

Making time for leisure is critical. Prioritizing relaxation, whether through hobbies, leisure activities, or just downtime, has a good impact on overall stress levels and sperm quality.

Environmental Factors Affecting Sperm Quality

Avoiding Toxins in the Environment

Chemical Exposure Reduction:

It is critical for sperm health to limit exposure to environmental contaminants like as pesticides, industrial chemicals, and pollution. Protective measures, such as wearing protective gear, help to reduce exposure.

Organic Product Selection:

Choosing organic items, particularly fruits and vegetables, decreases pesticide exposure. This deliberate choice contributes to a cleaner, toxin-free environment for sperm production.

Limiting Endocrine Disruptor Exposure

Chemicals that disrupt the endocrine system:

Endocrine disruptors, which can be found in certain plastics, home products, and personal care products, can disturb hormonal balance. It is critical for reproductive health to choose goods that are free of these disruptors.

BPA-Free Items:

Bisphenol A (BPA) has been identified as an endocrine disruptor. Using BPA-free goods, such as food containers and water bottles, lowers exposure and promotes hormonal balance.

Habits That Affect Sperm Quality

Quitting Smoking

The Effects of Smoking on Sperm:

Smoking is linked to lower sperm count, motility, and morphology. Quitting smoking is a critical step toward better sperm quality and reproductive health.

Smoking Cessation Assistance Programs:

Participating in smoking cessation programs or getting help from healthcare professionals increases the chances of quitting successfully.

These programs provide resources and tactics for quitting smoking.

Moderation with alcohol

The Effects of Alcohol on Sperm:

Excessive alcohol consumption might have an adverse effect on hormonal balance and sperm quality. Alcohol consumption in moderation or abstinence promotes a better reproductive environment.

Limits Establishment:

Setting clear limitations on alcohol usage is critical. Understanding individual tolerance and selecting non-alcoholic options benefits reproductive health.

Supplements that Improve Sperm Quality

Coenzyme Q10 (CoQ10) is a type of antioxidant.

CoQ10's Function:

Coenzyme Q10 is an antioxidant that helps the mitochondria operate properly. Supplementing with CoQ10 may improve sperm motility and protect against oxidative damage.

Selecting Ubiquinol:

Ubiquinol is the most absorbable active form of CoQ10. Choosing ubiquinol supplements ensures optimal efficacy in promoting sperm quality.

Acetyl-L-Carnitine and L-Carnitine

Sperm Motility Aid:

Acetyl-L-Carnitine and L-Carnitine are amino acids that help sperm motility. These supplements can help those who want to improve the mobility of their sperm.

Formulas for Combinations:

Certain supplements contain numerous substances, such as L-Carnitine and Acetyl-L-Carnitine, to provide comprehensive sperm quality support. Combination formulations may provide synergistic benefits.

Fertility testing and professional advice

Consultation with an andrologist

Andrologists' Role:

Andrologists, or male reproductive health professionals, are critical in assessing and managing sperm quality issues. Consulting with an andrologist ensures a full evaluation and tailored recommendations.

Collaborative Fertility Assessment:

Fertility testing is frequently a team effort involving both couples. Consultations with reproductive endocrinologists and fertility specialists help to provide a complete picture of the fertility landscape.

Analysis and Testing of Sperm

Parameters for Semen Analysis:

Semen analysis evaluates important factors such as sperm count, motility, and morphology. Understanding the findings of sperm analysis informs subsequent evaluation and treatment options.

Monitoring on a regular basis:

Regular sperm analysis provides insight into progress for individuals actively attempting to improve sperm quality. This monitoring aids in the refinement of tactics and the tailoring of treatments as needed.

Medical Treatments to Improve Sperm Quality

Hormonal Treatments

Taking Care of Hormonal Imbalances:

Hormonal abnormalities that affect sperm quality can be treated using hormonal treatments. These treatments are intended to restore hormonal balance and promote optimum spermatogenesis.

Replacement Therapy for Testosterone:

When testosterone levels are low, testosterone replacement therapy may be considered. This treatment promotes hormonal balance and reproductive health in general.

Surgical Procedures

Repair of Varicocele:

Varicoceles, or swollen veins in the scrotum, can have an effect on sperm quality. The goal of varicocele surgery is to enhance blood flow and create a better environment for sperm development.

Surgery for Reconstruction:

Reconstructive surgery may be recommended in cases when blockages or anatomical abnormalities are impeding sperm transmission. These techniques are designed to address specific issues impacting sperm motility.

Holistic Methods for Improving Sperm Quality

Mind-Body Relationship

Meditation and mindfulness:
Mindfulness techniques and meditation help to reduce stress and support the mind-body connection. These methods have a good impact on general well-being, including reproductive health.

Yoga as a Fertility Aid:

Yoga incorporates physical postures, breath control, and meditation. Yoga techniques designed specifically for fertility help to maintain hormonal balance and improve reproductive health.

Reproductive Health Acupuncture

Approach to Traditional Chinese Medicine:
Acupuncture, which has its roots in ancient Chinese medicine, is thought to balance the body's energy flow. Acupuncture may improve sperm quality and reproductive outcomes, according to some research.

Consultation with Practitioners of Traditional Chinese Medicine:
Acupuncture for reproductive assistance should be discussed with an expert traditional Chinese

medicine practitioner. Individualized therapies can be provided by these providers.

A Path to Better Fertility

The enhancement of sperm quality is a key step in the quest for motherhood, delicately knit into the fabric of reproductive health. This thorough resource provides a road map for men and couples navigating the complex terrain of male fertility.

The path to improved sperm quality is diverse, ranging from eating a nutrient-rich diet and making lifestyle changes to seeking professional advice and investigating holistic techniques. As individuals and couples embark on this life-changing journey, may the collective wisdom contained in these ideas illuminate the way forward, inspiring hope, resilience, and the

realization of the common desire of welcoming
new life.

CHAPTER 7

Medical Interventions

Assisted Reproductive Technologies (ART)

In the field of fertility, where the path to motherhood may present particular problems, the introduction of Assisted Reproductive Technologies (ART) has transformed the landscape, providing hope and chances for individuals and couples attempting to start families. This in-depth investigation digs into the complex realm of ART, unraveling the myriad technology, processes, ethical concerns, and emotional terrain that accompany this revolutionary approach to conception.

Learning About Assisted Reproductive Technologies (ART)

ART DEFINITION

ART refers to a wide range of medical techniques meant to help individuals or couples get pregnant. These technologies interfere with the natural process of pregnancy, providing options for persons with infertility or reproductive difficulties.

ART's Scope:

ART comprises a variety of procedures in addition to in vitro fertilization (IVF), such as intrauterine insemination (IUI), gamete intrafallopian transfer (GIFT), and intracytoplasmic sperm injection (ICSI). Each approach targets a different part of reproductive difficulties.

IUI stands for intrauterine insemination.

Overview of the Process:

During the ovulatory phase, sperm is directly introduced into the woman's uterus. This approach allows sperm to be closer to the egg, improving the likelihood of fertilization.

Indications for IUI include:

IUI is typically advised for couples experiencing unexplained infertility, minor male factor infertility, or cervical problems that may prevent spontaneous conception. When compared to more complex ART techniques, it is a less invasive choice.

IVF stands for In Vitro Fertilization.

IVF in a Nutshell:

IVF is a well-known and extensively used ART treatment. It entails removing eggs from the ovaries, fertilizing them with sperm in a laboratory dish, and transferring the resulting embryos into the uterus.

Indications for IVF include:

IVF is used to treat a variety of fertility issues, including tubal factor infertility, endometriosis, male factor infertility, and unexplained infertility. It is frequently considered when other reproductive therapies have failed.

Gamete Intrafallopian Transfer (GIFT)

GIFT Methodology:

GIFT entails the harvesting of eggs, sperm, and possibly embryos, which are subsequently put into the fallopian tubes immediately. Fertilization takes place naturally within the female reproductive system.

GIFT justification:

Individuals or couples with intact fallopian tubes and a preference for fertilization to occur within the body rather than in a laboratory setting may benefit from GIFT. It is a less prevalent ART technique nowadays.

ICSI stands for Intracytoplasmic Sperm Injection.

ICSI Procedure:

ICSI is a procedure that involves injecting a single sperm directly into an egg to induce conception. This approach is especially beneficial in cases of male factor infertility, where sperm quantity or quality may be a limiting factor.

ICSI Applications:

When standard IVF is ineffective owing to severe male factor infertility, ICSI is used. It has been shown to be effective in cases of low sperm count, poor sperm motility, or sperm morphological problems.

Donor Sperm and Egg

Using Donor Eggs:

Donor eggs may be a viable alternative for individuals or couples experiencing difficulties with egg quality or ovarian function. This entails taking donor eggs, fertilizing them with sperm, and then transferring the resulting embryos to the recipient's uterus.

Overview of Sperm Donation:

Sperm donation is an option for men who have severe male factor infertility and whose sperm is unsuitable for conception. Donor sperm can be utilized in ART treatments such as IUI and IVF.

Surrogacy

Surrogacy Explained:

Surrogacy is the use of a gestational carrier to carry and deliver a baby for individuals or couples who are unable to carry their own pregnancy. The surrogate has no genetic connection to the child.

Surrogacy Types:

The most frequent type is gestational surrogacy, in which the surrogate carries an embryo generated from the intended parents' or donors' gametes. In traditional surrogacy, the surrogate provides both the egg and the pregnancy.

PGT stands for Preimplantation Genetic Testing.

PGT's Purpose:

PGT is a series of genetic tests performed on embryos prior to implantation into the uterus during IVF. Its goal is to find genetic anomalies, chromosomal problems, and specific genetic ailments.

PGT classifications:

PGT is divided into three types: PGT-A (aneuploidy screening), PGT-M (monogenic/single gene diseases), and PGT-SR (structural rearrangements). Each kind has a specific function in determining the genetic health of embryos.

Ethical Issues in Assisted Reproductive Technology

Selection and Disposition of Embryos

Ethical Issues in PGT:

The ability to choose embryos using genetic factors poses ethical concerns. The selection process, potential consequences for the child's identity, and the disposition of unused embryos are all major ethical quandaries.

Autonomy and Responsibility in Balance:

The difficulty of ART is to strike a balance between individual autonomy and the duty of making decisions that consider the well-being of future children. Ethical guidelines attempt to handle these difficult situations.

Donor Identity and Conception

Identity Investigation:

Individuals conceived using donor eggs or sperm may face identity and genetic heritage issues. Individuals' right to know their genetic origins is one of the ethical considerations.

Donor Relationship Openness:

Practices that promote transparency in donor-conceived interactions, such as revealing donor information or facilitating communication if requested, contribute to donor conception ethics.

Access to and Commercialization of Art

Economic Aspects of ART:

The economic implications of ART, such as the cost of surgeries, drugs, and associated medical bills, present ethical issues. Access to fertility treatments should ideally be equal, with no financial constraints limiting reproductive options.

Global Inequalities:

Global disparities in ART access occur, with variances in availability, price, and legal regulations. Addressing global gaps and advocating for equitable reproductive healthcare are both ethical considerations.

ART's Emotional and Psychological Dimensions

Treatment's Influence on Mental Health

Emotional Highs and Lows:

The ART journey can be emotionally exhausting, with highs of hope and lows of disappointment. Understanding and managing the psychological impact of reproductive treatments is critical for individual and couple well-being.

Adaptation Mechanisms:

Individuals can negotiate the emotional complications of fertility treatments by developing appropriate coping skills, such as obtaining support from mental health specialists, support groups, or therapy.

Informed Consent and Decision-Making

Making Informed Decisions:

Informed consent is a key component of ethical ART practice. Individuals and couples can make more educated decisions if they are given thorough information regarding treatments, dangers, success rates, and potential results.

Making Decisions Together:

Open communication between healthcare practitioners and patients is required for collaborative decision-making. Individuals and couples that use shared decision-making actively participate in selecting the course of their fertility journey.

ART Legal Considerations

Rights and Responsibilities of Parents

Creating Parental Rights:

In cases of ART, legal frameworks differ in determining parental rights and obligations. Legal agreements, especially those involving surrogacy or the use of donor gametes, must be clear in order to safeguard the rights of all parties involved.

Surrogacy Laws Around the World:

Surrogacy regulations vary greatly among countries, creating complications when individuals or couples seek surrogacy agreements on a global scale. Understanding and navigating these legal landscapes is critical for a legal and successful surrogacy process.

Future ART Trends and Advancements

Technological Advances

Reproductive Science Advances:

Ongoing research and technology advancements continue to transform the ART scene. Emerging technologies, such as AI applications in embryo selection and CRISPR gene editing, bring both opportunities and ethical concerns.

Increasing Success Rates:

Continued attempts to improve procedures, laboratory settings, and understanding of reproductive biology all lead to higher ART success rates. Ongoing research promises to make greater advances in the subject.

The Changing Face of Family Formation

Assisted Reproductive Technologies exist as a tribute to human inventiveness and the unwavering desire for parenting in the ever-changing world of family building. ART provides a range of alternatives, from intrauterine insemination to preimplantation genetic testing and beyond, each with its own set of considerations and opportunities.

Individuals and couples must approach the complexity of fertility treatments with informed decision-making, emotional resilience, and a deep grasp of the ethical issues involved. The route to parenting via ART is intensely personal and transformative, marked by optimism, struggles, and the extraordinary promise for fresh beginnings. May this exploration serve as a guide, throwing light on the many elements of Assisted Reproductive Technologies and providing education, compassion, and steadfast support to individuals on the journey to motherhood.

Treatments and Options for Fertility

The path to parenthood is a very personal and changing event. The landscape of fertility treatments and options opens doors to new possibilities for individuals and couples who are having difficulty conceiving naturally. This detailed resource guides readers through numerous medical interventions, outlining the various ways available to people looking to start a family.

Understanding Fertility Issues

Infertility Definition

Infertility Explained:

The failure to conceive after a year of regular, unprotected intercourse is typically classified as infertility. It can affect both men and women and be caused by a variety of circumstances such as hormonal imbalances, structural difficulties, or reproductive health issues.

Infertility, Primary and Secondary:

Primary infertility is the inability to have a first child, whereas secondary infertility happens when a couple struggles to conceive after previously conceiving.

The First Steps in Fertility Evaluation

Diagnostic Testing

Complete Medical History:

The first stage in fertility assessment is a detailed medical history to discover potential causes of infertility. Exploration of reproductive health, menstrual history, sexual history, and any pre-existing medical issues is included.

Physical Examiners:

Physical examinations, such as pelvic examinations for women and sperm analysis for males, provide important information on reproductive health. Further diagnostic assessments are guided by identifying any physical anomalies or concerns.

Fundamental Fertility Treatments

Induction of Ovulation

Increasing Egg Production:

Ovulation induction is the use of drugs to stimulate the ovaries and increase egg production, such as Clomiphene citrate or gonadotropins. This method is advantageous for women who have irregular ovulation.

Ovulation Tracking:

Monitoring during ovulation induction include tracking hormone levels and performing ultrasound scans to observe follicle development. To improve chances of conception, timed intercourse or intrauterine insemination (IUI) may be recommended.

Fertility Treatments of the Future

IUI stands for intrauterine insemination.

Controlling Sperm Placement:

During the ovulatory phase, sperm is directly placed into the woman's uterus. This treatment increases the likelihood of fertilization by bringing sperm closer to the egg.

Indications for IUI include:

IUI is frequently advised for couples experiencing unexplained infertility, minor male factor infertility, or cervical problems that may prevent spontaneous conception. When compared to more advanced reproductive treatments, it is a less invasive choice.

IVF stands for In Vitro Fertilization.

Fertilization and Egg Harvesting:

IVF is a popular fertility therapy that involves removing eggs from the ovaries, fertilizing them in a laboratory dish with sperm, and transferring the resulting embryos into the uterus.

Indications for IVF include:

IVF is used to treat infertility issues such as tubal factor infertility, endometriosis, male factor infertility, and unexplained infertility. It is frequently prescribed when other reproductive therapies have failed.

ICSI stands for Intracytoplasmic Sperm Injection.

Injection of Sperm Directly:

ICSI is a type of IVF in which a single sperm is directly inserted into an egg to aid in fertilization. This method is very useful in cases of severe male factor infertility.

ICSI Applications:

ICSI is used when standard IVF may be ineffective due to issues such as low sperm count, poor sperm motility, or sperm morphological defects.

Donor sperm and eggs

Using Donor Eggs:

Donor eggs may be a viable alternative for individuals or couples experiencing difficulties with egg quality or ovarian function. This entails taking donor eggs, fertilizing them with sperm, and then transferring the resulting embryos to the recipient's uterus.

Overview of Sperm Donation:

Sperm donation is an option for men who have severe male factor infertility and whose sperm is unsuitable for conception. Donor sperm can be utilized in reproductive procedures such as IUI and IVF.

Surrogacy

Making Use of a Gestational Carrier:

Surrogacy is the use of a gestational carrier to carry and deliver a baby for individuals or couples who are unable to carry their own pregnancy. The surrogate has no genetic connection to the child.

Surrogacy Types:

The most frequent type is gestational surrogacy, in which the surrogate carries an embryo generated from the intended parents' or donors' gametes. In traditional surrogacy, the surrogate provides both the egg and the pregnancy.

PGT stands for Preimplantation Genetic Testing.

PGT's Purpose:

PGT is a series of genetic tests performed on embryos prior to implantation into the uterus during IVF. Its goal is to find genetic anomalies, chromosomal problems, and specific genetic ailments.

PGT classifications:

PGT is divided into three types: PGT-A (aneuploidy screening), PGT-M (monogenic/single gene diseases), and PGT-SR (structural rearrangements). Each kind has a specific function in determining the genetic health of embryos.

Fertility Treatments That Are Holistic

Changes in Lifestyle

Exercise and nutrition:

Adopting a balanced and nutritious diet rich in vital vitamins and minerals benefits reproductive health overall. Regular exercise promotes hormonal balance and overall health.

Weight Control:

It is critical for fertility to maintain a healthy weight. Obesity and underweight can both have a deleterious impact on reproductive function. Achieving and maintaining a healthy weight increases the likelihood of conception.

Stress Reduction

The Effects of Stress on Fertility:

Chronic stress can interrupt menstrual periods by affecting reproductive hormones. Stress-reduction strategies such as meditation, yoga, or mindfulness increase emotional well-being and fertility.

Mind-Body Techniques:

Mind-body therapies, such as acupuncture and relaxation techniques, provide holistic approaches to stress management and improving the mind-body connection. These methods supplement traditional fertility treatments.

Alternative Medicine

Fertility Acupuncture:
Acupuncture, which has its roots in traditional Chinese medicine, is thought to aid conception by increasing energy balance and circulation. Acupuncture may be useful as a supplemental therapy during fertility treatments for certain people.

Supplements with herbs:
Certain herbal supplements may help with reproductive health. However, before

introducing herbal therapies into reproductive planning, it is critical to check with a healthcare expert because their safety and efficacy differ.

Managing Male Factor Infertility

Treatments for Male Fertility

Hormonal Treatments:

hormone imbalances that affect male fertility can be treated with hormone treatments. These treatments are intended to restore hormonal balance and promote healthy sperm production.

Surgical Procedures:

To address problems that contribute to male infertility, surgical procedures such as varicocele surgery or anatomical modifications may be indicated.

Preserving Fertility

Freezing eggs:

Women can preserve their eggs for future use by freezing them. This is advantageous for persons undergoing medical treatments that may have an influence on fertility or those who prefer to postpone childbearing for personal reasons.

Sperm donation:

Sperm banking allows men to preserve their fertility. This is frequently examined prior to medical treatments or operations that may have an impact on sperm production or quality.

Psychiatric Assistance During Fertility Treatments

Counseling Services and Support Groups:
Fertility treatments can have a profound emotional impact. Individuals and couples can

vent their emotions, share their experiences, and receive assistance through counseling and involvement in support groups.

Mind-Body Techniques:

Mind-body therapies, such as fertility yoga or meditation, combine psychological and physical well-being. These programs provide holistic approaches to dealing with stress and emotional difficulties.

Each thread in the rich tapestry of fertility treatments and options reflects a distinct approach, a specific obstacle, or a hopeful opportunity. Understanding the range of alternatives accessible to individuals and couples as they travel this path enables them to make informed decisions that are aligned with their objectives and values.

The path to parenthood is complex, ranging from basic therapies for individual fertility issues to modern assisted reproductive technologies. Holistic therapies, lifestyle changes, and emotional support supplement medical interventions, establishing a holistic approach to reproductive health.

May this book serve as a compass, highlighting the various paths that individuals and couples might take in their journey to start a family. May hope, resilience, and the collective wisdom of medical discoveries guide those on the journey to parenthood, fostering the fulfillment of goals and the delight of embracing new life with each step.

CHAPTER 8

Success Stories

Actual Life Experiences

Individual and couple real-life experiences navigating this route serve as powerful narratives, revealing the various ways people face and overcome barriers on the road to parenting. We dig into the victories, hardships, and unflinching tenacity that characterize the human experience of generating life in this investigation of real-life fertility stories.

Embracing the Emotional Rollercoaster

The First Struggle:

Disappointment at the Outset:

For many, the journey begins with hope and excitement, only to be followed by months of sadness as conception proves elusive. Each negative pregnancy test takes an emotional toll, and couples are frequently confronted with the unexpected weight of infertility.

The Decision to Seek Assistance:

Many individuals and couples seek expert help after discovering that their conception is not progressing as expected. The choice to visit fertility specialists is a watershed event, defined by a mix of hope, concern, and a determination to understand and address the underlying issues.

Starting Fertility Treatments:

The Initial Steps:

Fertility treatments, such as ovulation induction, intrauterine insemination (IUI), or in vitro fertilization (IVF), become a part of the journey for people interested in assisted reproductive technologies. The first steps into these treatments are frequently accompanied by a mixture of exhilaration and apprehension.

Uncertainty Management:

The unpredictable nature of reproductive treatments adds another element of uncertainty. Real-life stories depict the emotional rollercoaster of cycles that offer hope with each embryo transfer or IUI, only to be met with sadness when the results are negative.

Victories and Celebrations

Against the Odds Success:

The Pleasure of Positive Outcomes:
Real-life fertility stories are laced with triumphant moments in which couples overcome hurdles and enjoy great outcomes. Successful IVF cycles, overcoming male factor infertility, and conceiving against all odds all produce compelling stories of strength and determination.

Pregnancy Miracles:
Some stories depict pregnancies that can only be defined as miraculous. Natural conceptions after years of fertility treatments or unexpected pregnancies after a period of infertility treatment cessation demonstrate the unpredictability of the fertility journey.

Adoption and Family Formation:

Adoption Experiences:

Real-life experiences also include making the decision to start a family through adoption. Adoption stories, whether local or international, emphasize the various paths to parenting and the joy of establishing families through various means.

Blended Families and Unusual Pathways:

Blended families, in which individuals or couples bring children from past relationships together, and unusual avenues to parenthood, such as co-parenting arrangements or surrogacy, highlight the changing landscape of family formation.

Dealing with Obstacles and Difficulties

Managing Failed Treatments:

The Anguish of Failed Cycles:
Real-life fertility stories recognize the anguish of unsuccessful therapies. Couples frequently discuss the emotional toll of miscarriages, failed IVF cycles, or failed attempts at conception, emphasizing the strength required to overcome these failures.

Coping with the Loss of a Pregnancy:
Unfortunately, pregnancy loss is a regular element of the fertility quest. Real-life examples highlight the sadness, mourning, and emotional issues that individuals and couples encounter following miscarriages, highlighting the significance of emotional support during these trying times.

Relationship Effects:

Understanding Relationship Dynamics:
Even the strongest relationships can be tested during the reproductive process. Real-life accounts openly examine the impact of fertility issues on relationships, examining how couples manage the emotional highs and lows while remaining communicative and supportive of one another.

Seeking Counseling and Assistance:
Many accounts emphasize the critical function of counseling and support groups in assisting couples to traverse the emotional turmoil. Seeking professional help becomes an important part of the process, offering strategies to cope with stress, sorrow, and interpersonal difficulties.

Personal Development and Transformation

Finding Strength in Adversity:

Accepting Vulnerability:

Real-life fertility stories frequently demonstrate the strength that may be discovered in vulnerability. Couples and individuals openly express their hardships, creating a feeling of community and breaking down stigmas associated with infertility. This transparency helps to foster a culture of support and understanding.

Sharing Leads to Empowerment:

Individuals and couples who share their personal experiences are better able to advocate for their needs and make educated decisions. Real-life tales serve as change agents, motivating others to get treatment, prioritize their mental health, and tackle the reproductive journey with tenacity.

Finding Resilience:

Resilience Revealed:

The fertility journey demonstrates individuals' and couples' tremendous perseverance. There are several examples of people overcoming adversity, confronting setbacks head on, and rising from difficulties with greater strength and drive.

Perspective Changes:

Real-life events frequently result in major alterations in viewpoint. Individuals and couples discuss how the reproductive journey, with all of its ups and downs, promotes reevaluations of priorities, aspirations, and family definitions, resulting in dramatic personal growth.

Conceiving can be difficult for certain couples; approximately 9% of men and 11% of women are stated to have a reproductive problem that prevents or makes conception difficult. When you add a chronic health issue to the mix, things can get much more complicated.

According to several studies, a variety of chronic diseases, ranging from heart disease to diabetes, can inhibit both ovulation and sperm production, making it harder to become pregnant. Thyroid problems can interfere with ovulation. Treatments for cancer, such as chemotherapy and radiation, might impair fertility. According to research, several autoimmune disorders, such as lupus and rheumatoid arthritis, may impair your ability to start a family.

Listen to Their Stories

Name: Lisa,

Age: 42

Profession: Relationship Counselor

Location: Washington, D.C.

Fertility Battle: Trying to conceive with undiagnosed celiac disease, an immunological response to gluten present in meals containing wheat, barley, and rye.

Lisa experienced a miscarriage in her early forties before becoming pregnant and taking her baby to term. Lisa experienced two further miscarriages over the next few years, both of which were distressing, including one that resulted in a bacterial infection in her uterus that went misdiagnosed for nearly a year. Despite being physically and emotionally exhausted as a result of these events, she and her husband sought to expand their family.

"I saw a fertility doctor and he ran a battery of blood tests, including an antibody test," Lisa said. "Running the antibody test is not standard practice, but it suggested I had celiac [disease]." I didn't have digestion issues, but I was suffering from severe migraines in the middle of the night and headaches at the base of my skull all day. The headaches disappeared as soon as I stopped eating gluten. I felt more relaxed and less emotional. And, later on, I realized [how] rapid my digestion had been, and it slowed down."

"My doctor encouraged me to try a round of IVF right away," she continues, because she'd already experienced three miscarriages. "I spoke with a gastroenterologist, who told me that once the gluten was out of my system, my body would respond better." If I wasn't receiving nourishment, neither was the baby."

Several studies have identified a link between celiac disease and infertility, implying that between 4% and 8% of women with infertility have gluten sensitivity. The reasons are unknown, but experts believe systemic inflammation or nutrition absorption issues may be at blame. What's the good news? According to a study of 11,000 Swedish women, fertility is commonly recovered after diagnosis and treatment (following a rigorous gluten-free diet).

"I remember thinking my body needs time to rest and heal," she recalls. "However, the fertility doctors said, 'Don't wait six months.'" And because of insurance and time, we could practically perform a round of IVF for free, so we did. My energy wasn't there. I blew it. I didn't say anything. I only laid one egg. I did not become pregnant. I had a complete breakdown. I traveled to France and smoked and drank the entire time. "I was sick of trying so hard."

Lisa began visiting a fertility coach, who provides tailored and holistic support on the path to parenthood. Fertility coaches, like other forms of health coaches, vary in their accreditations. Some provide comprehensive nutritional and lifestyle guidance. Others provide specialized treatment advice, while still others focus on emotional support and therapy. The coach's style is determined by his or her education and background, which might range from registered nurse to licensed therapist to acupuncturist to no credentials at all. Keep in mind that there is no standard certification method, professional oversight, or licensure for fertility coaches. Lisa says she met her fertility coach at her acupuncture clinic, which she visits "religiously." Acupuncture has long been used as an alternative fertility treatment, however medical investigations have yielded inconsistent outcomes.

"I remember telling [my coach] that the fertility process felt all or nothing—that I could do acupuncture and try more fertility treatments, or I could be done." She helped me realize how much I was willing to do and that it could be enough. I was sick of running around to acupuncture appointments. I didn't want to stop drinking or exercising. Someone suggested I consult a Chinese herbalist. That sounded like something I'd be willing to do. As a result, I went. She told me my system was depleted and made this tea from dried flowers and roots for me. The tea stinked up the entire home, yet I could feel it warming and feeding my insides."

Her coach also assisted her in focusing on what she already had rather than mourning what she felt to be lacking, she says. "We concentrated on what was working in my life, noticing it and being grateful for it." My husband and I began to re-orient ourselves and reflect on our lovely life with our one child. A month later, I discovered I was pregnant—with twins. The pregnancy was really difficult, and I spent the entire time certain that it was all a dream. But the twins have arrived."

What I wish I'd known: "As women, we put so much pressure on ourselves. It's as if we have to prove how much we want the baby in order to deserve it. It's all too simple to push yourself beyond your comfort zone. It's tempting to believe that if I don't do everything, I don't deserve this baby in some way. That is simply not the case. My coach assisted me in navigating this, determining what I was comfortable with and being at peace with it. It was extremely beneficial, and I cannot suggest it highly enough."

Name: Alison

Age: 46

Profession: Psychiatrist

Location: Middletown, New York

Fertility Battle: Pursuing a "geriatric" pregnancy (when the pregnant person is 35 or older) with uterine fibroids (UF), which are benign but often bothersome growths, and endometriosis, a disorder in which endometrial tissue grows beyond the uterine lining. Both disorders can cause extremely painful menstrual cycles and problems conceiving.

Alison was diagnosed with UF as a teenager, followed by endometriosis in her twenties. Heavy periods, strong cramps, and discomfort caused her to double over and miss class on a regular basis throughout college. Alison had many procedures for both throughout her twenties and understood that getting pregnant might be tough one day.

"I got married in 2008 and started seeing a fertility specialist right away," said Alison. "They tested my egg reserve and discovered that I had a good, healthy number." I wanted to enjoy myself, so when I asked my doctor if I could wait a year, he agreed."

However, just 12 months later, they examined her again and discovered that her egg count had dropped by half. Alison was compelled to take action and began fertility treatments, beginning with tubal flushing, in which doctors blasted dye into the fallopian tubes to clear any obstructions and create a passage for the sperm to travel through. Alison became pregnant right away after the treatment—the only time she did so naturally—but the pregnancy terminated in miscarriage.

"Everything was really emotional. I was seeing the pregnancies of my pals. I have a cousin who refuses to speak to me because I did not accompany her to the hospital when her son was born. It was around the time I would have been due had I not miscarried. And I couldn't do it. I simply couldn't."

Alison turned to IVF at that point. "I got pregnant, but it ended with an ectopic pregnancy," which occurs when the fertilized egg implants outside of the womb, most commonly in the fallopian tube. "They gave me birth control pills to end the pregnancy." One of my fallopian tubes was removed. After a month, doctors determined that I was at high risk for another [ectopic pregnancy] and removed the tube."

Alison still had eggs even when her tubes were gone. Alison and her husband were heartbroken after a second round of IVF failed to produce any viable eggs. "You're going through emotional pain, physical pain, and now financial pain due to a third round of IVF that isn't covered by insurance." I became pregnant on the third try, but my beta HCG levels [a pregnancy hormone] were not increasing as expected, and the doctors couldn't [detect] the heartbeat. They didn't think the pregnancy was viable and advised me to terminate it due of my history."

Alison says she was so upset by the news that she couldn't drive herself home. "I went with my parents to this [appointment] because my husband was away." I informed my doctor that I couldn't make the decision [to terminate the pregnancy] without first consulting with him. I also realized I couldn't go on like this. I was a nervous wreck. I went home and drank some wine."

But her doctors were mistaken, and she's glad she insisted on taking her time before having a D&C, a procedure that removes nonviable fetal tissue.

"I put my name on a bunch of adoption waiting lists," Alison recalls. "I returned to my doctor, and they did an ultrasound just to be sure." The baby's heartbeat was really strong. My doctor expressed cautious optimism. I was still in shambles. I kept my pregnancy a secret from everyone. I couldn't stop crying. I wouldn't let my mother throw me a baby shower until two weeks before my C-section. My baby was fine when she was delivered, but I was still a wreck. I suffered a slight bowel obstruction, a tube down my nose, and spent an extra week in the hospital. But my miraculous Malbec baby is already eight years old."

What I wish I had known: "It's a difficult, lonely process." My family was quite supportive, but half of my friends had no idea I was pregnant. There was also a limit to how much I wanted to [discuss with] my mother or husband—I kept far too much to myself. I was afraid that if I got too excited, I'd jinx it and something would go wrong. It would have been beneficial to speak with someone who has gone through this before. I was aware of the medical aspect of it. I had the answers from the book, but not the actual knowledge. It's a huge emotional drain. It would have been far better if I had sought assistance or gone through some counseling. According to the psychiatrist, I should have seen a therapist!"

Name: Lin

Age: 35

Profession: Stylist

Location: Newport, Rhode Island

Fertility Battle: Trying to conceive with polycystic ovarian syndrome (PCOS), a hormonal disease that causes tiny fluid-filled sacs to grow on the ovaries. Infertility can result from the disorder, which can cause irregular periods, pelvic pain, and infertility.

Lin was diagnosed with PCOS when she was a teenager and was put on birth control to manage her symptoms. She wasn't concerned about fertility at the moment, given her youthful age. And when she was ready to have a baby, her physicians assured her that "it will probably be fine."

"My husband and I had been married for a few years and decided to start trying," Lin adds. "When I stopped taking the Pill, my body freaked out." My menstrual cycles were irregular. I was losing hair. "I was gaining weight for no apparent reason."

It turned out that the birth control was disguising an underlying and undetected health issue—but it would take months for her and her fertility team to figure out what was going on.

Her doctors first analyzed her estrogen, progesterone, prolactin, and other hormone levels, which she was informed were all normal. "I pushed back and said, 'I don't have a period, and that's not normal.'" I was referred to a reproductive endocrinologist. I felt like I was working on a factory farm after I got there. You go in, have bloodwork, and then follow these exact instructions. Everyone seems to get the same steps, no matter what's going on—and you're continually poked and prodded."

But, she adds, that's not all. She was put on letrozole, a cancer medicine that can be used for fertility off-label. According to a study published in Frontiers in Endocrinology, the medicine decreases estrogen levels, so when you stop taking it, you experience a rush of estrogen and follicle growth. "I did it three times in one month," Lin says. "I was exhausted and emotional." There's also the added pressure of having sex on a timetable. It's not coming from a fun or exciting place; there's an element of force about it."

On top of that, the COVID pandemic was raging, leaving the nurses tired. "My reproductive endocrinologist was nice, but the staff was terrible," Lin said. "When they called, it was as if they hadn't even looked at my chart. To be treated so casually added to my annoyance... One nurse told me I shouldn't try to get pregnant since we don't know how COVID affects newborns yet. There was always the possibility that we might be shut down."

Lin was obliged to perform routine bloodwork and ultrasounds alone due to pandemic limitations; her spouse was not permitted to accompany her. "It was quite alienating... I needed a break after a month of that. It was dreadful."

That's when she discovered a PCOS-specific registered dietician. "I began better balancing my meals, drinking more water, and moving differently." I was spinning three times per week. And I discovered that my body perceives that as a stressor and releases all of this cortisol." While research on exercise and fertility is conflicting, it appears that while exercise is beneficial, high amounts of intensive activity may affect fertility. Furthermore, when trying to conceive, research indicates that severe exercise be limited to no more than four hours per week, with no need to limit moderate exercise. Although it is unknown if strenuous exercise produces enough cortisol to affect fertility, studies does show that chronic stress can damage conception.

Lin had a DUTCH test, a costly procedure that evaluates hormone-metabolite levels in dried urine but has not been validated in independent research and is rarely utilized by traditional doctors' offices. Lin, on the other hand, claims to have discovered that her body was not processing insulin properly. She was warned she was predisposed to type 2 diabetes and heart problems. "That was game-changing." I did more research and discovered that those who took letrozole first may have [fertility] success. I had to fight hard for myself to get metformin." She continues. "We did two rounds of a metformin-letrozole combination, and the second time I got pregnant." We now have an eight-month-old."

What I wish I'd known prior to my pregnancy: "Having a more well-rounded approach and thinking about my fertility journey as a whole-mind, whole-body experience was huge,"

Lin tells me. "Some people would like you to meditate. Others want you to do medical things and take medicines. I took the judgments that felt right for me and drew inspiration from everywhere. It would be extremely beneficial if you could join a support group... That made me feel less alone in this."

Getting to the Heart of Science and Hope

Science and Technology's Role:

Utilizing Technological Advances:

Actual fertility anecdotes highlight the importance of scientific advances in assisted reproduction technology. Individuals and couples express thanks for the chances provided by these technologies, which range from advancements in IVF to revolutionary genetic testing tools.

Fertility Science is Changing:

A frequent theme in narratives is the changing environment of fertility science. Individuals and couples discuss their experiences with developing treatments, emphasizing the field's continual growth and the hope it has for future generations.

Hope and Realism in Balance:

The Difficult Balance:

Real-life examples demonstrate the delicate balance that people and couples must strike between hope and realism. Managing expectations, accepting uncertainty, and enjoying minor achievements all become important components of the reproductive journey.

Hope as a Motivator:

In fertility stories, hope emerges as a significant motivating force. Individuals and couples are sustained through the ups and downs of the journey by their everlasting belief in the potential of motherhood, despite hurdles and failures.

Hope, Resilience, and New Beginnings Stories

Each story in the mosaic of real-life fertility stories adds to a communal fabric of hope, resilience, and the enduring human spirit. These stories go beyond medical jargon to show the very emotional and transforming aspect of the fertility experience.

Individuals and couples who share their stories not only navigate their own pathways, but also pave the way for others who are traveling a similar path. Real-life fertility experiences demonstrate that while each person's journey to motherhood is unique, the threads of hope, resilience, and the quest of family weave a common thread that ties us all.

May these stories serve as beacons of hope for people facing infertility issues, providing solace, understanding, and the knowledge that inside each narrative lies the possibility of fresh beginnings, joy, and the fulfillment of aspirations.

Overcoming Fertility Obstacles

Stories of overcoming obstacles serve as beacons of perseverance, dedication, and hope in the intricate fabric of the reproductive journey. Individuals and couples travel the maze of infertility, which is distinguished by twists, turns, and unforeseen detours, and emerge triumphant despite the odds. We delve into real-life success stories in this exploration, revealing the various ways people overcome fertility issues, establishing a feeling of community, and inspiring those on similar roads.

Accepting an Unpredictable Journey

The Uncharted Road:

A Journey Begins:

Each fertility journey begins with a blank canvas, ready to be painted with the colors of hope, endurance, and unyielding determination. Success tales frequently begin with the recognition that the path ahead is unpredictable, with its own set of challenges and victories.

Uncertainty Management:

Overcoming fertility issues entails navigating through unknowns. Couples discuss their experiences embracing the unexpected nature of the journey, responding to setbacks, and being committed to the ultimate goal of starting a family.

Victories amidst Setbacks

Managing Failed Cycles:

Resilience and Heartbreak:

Real-life success tales create resilience narratives in the face of failed cycles. Couples share their anguish from failed attempts and how they funneled that pain into greater determination, paving the door for following achievements.

Perseverance Lessons:

Perseverance emerges as a frequent motif in stories about breaking out from failing cycles. Couples frequently describe how setbacks turned into stepping stones, providing significant lessons and insights that spurred them further on their reproductive journey.

Experiencing Pregnancy Loss:

Grief and Recovery:

The heartbreaking experience of pregnancy loss can occasionally mark the path to parenting. Success stories dive into the subsequent pain, mourning, and healing, demonstrating the courage required to navigate the emotional intricacies while pursuing parenting.

Recovery after Loss:

Individuals and couples explain how they emerged stronger from the shadows of loss, demonstrating resilience. achievement stories demonstrate the transformative potential of transforming grief into a driving force that propels people toward newfound hope and eventual achievement.

Understanding Relationship Dynamics

Partnership Development:

The Influence on Relationships:

Even the strongest relationships can be tested by infertility. Success stories examine the impact of fertility issues on relationships, emphasizing the importance of open communication, mutual support, and link strengthening in the midst of emotional upheaval.

Mutual Development:

Couples share common growth stories, acknowledging that the fertility journey is a shared experience. Overcoming obstacles becomes a team effort, cultivating a deeper knowledge of one another and setting the groundwork for the future.

Seeking Assistance:

Counseling and Public Spaces:

Success stories emphasize the necessity of receiving expert assistance and participating in support groups. Counseling gave tools for couples to negotiate emotional tension, while support groups provided shared spaces for vulnerability, understanding, and encouragement.

Making Decisions Together:

Navigating fertility issues necessitates collaborative decision-making. Success tales show how couples actively participated in charting their own path, building a sense of agency and unity in the face of adversity.

Finding Unexpected Routes

Adoption Experiences:

Accepting Adoption:

For some, resolving fertility issues leads to an acceptance of adoption. Success stories highlight the transformative experiences of individuals and couples who found joy in starting families via adoption, emphasizing the richness of various paths to motherhood.

Blended Families and Unusual Pathways:
Real-life stories go beyond traditional narratives, with blended families and unusual paths to fatherhood. These stories depict the changing terrain of family formation, underlining that success in the reproductive journey can take numerous shapes.

Surprising Miracles:

Natural Thoughts Following Treatment:

In many success tales, miraculous pregnancies occur unexpectedly. Couples express their delight at conceiving naturally after years of fertility treatments, demonstrating that the most unexpected pathways may lead to the most profound victories.

Unexpected Pregnancies:

Some accounts involve unexpected pregnancies following periods of infertility treatment discontinuation. These unexpected turns highlight the erratic character of the fertility journey, reminding individuals and couples that hope can appear in unexpected ways.

Holistic Wellness Approaches

Changes in Lifestyle:

Exercise and nutrition:

Success stories frequently include lifestyle changes such as balanced meals and regular exercise. These modifications improve overall reproductive health, emphasizing the importance of holistic approaches to the fertility journey.

Holistic Wellness Techniques:

Adopting holistic wellness methods becomes a recurring theme in success tales. Couples discuss how disciplines like mindfulness, yoga, and acupuncture aided their mental well-being and increased fertility.

Alternative Medicine:

Acupuncture and herbal remedies:

Real-life success stories investigate the use of complementary therapies such as acupuncture and herbal supplements. Individuals and couples discuss how these old traditions-based approaches supplemented current therapy and contributed to their success.

The Mind-Body Connection

In success stories, the mind-body connection appears as a recurring motif. Meditation and relaxation activities are praised for their beneficial effects on stress reduction and overall well-being during the reproductive journey.

Celebrating Science's Role

Technological Progress:

Thanks to Assisted Reproductive Technologies:

Success stories show a deep appreciation for assisted reproductive technology. Individuals and couples highlight the significance of science in expanding possibilities and fulfilling ambitions, ranging from discoveries in IVF to revolutionary genetic testing techniques.

Fertility Science is Changing:

The changing landscape of fertility science demonstrates the tenacity of those who face difficulties. Success stories share their experiences with new treatments, demonstrating the field's ongoing advancement and the hope it instills in people on the reproductive path.

Hope and Realism in Balance:

Hope as a Motivator:

Success tales highlight the delicate mix between hope and realism. Individuals and couples discuss how keeping optimism, especially in the face of uncertainty, acts as a driving force in their journey to parenting.

Small Victories to Celebrate:

Real-life stories stress the importance of recognizing and enjoying minor triumphs along the way. Success is characterized not only by great achievements, but also by the perseverance displayed in overcoming each obstacle, no matter how minor.

Victory and New Beginnings

Success tales weave a tapestry of triumph, tenacity, and the unshakable human spirit in the vast landscape of reproductive issues. Each story is a distinct thread that contributes to a larger story of hope and inspiration for people embarking on or managing their own reproductive journeys.

May these stories serve as a reminder of the human capacity to overcome adversity. Every story of overcoming fertility issues contains a ray of hope, illuminating the path for others to achieve strength, perseverance, and the fulfillment of their ambitions.

CONCLUSION

We've traveled a complex tapestry of issues in this comprehensive investigation of fertility, each adding to a nuanced understanding of reproductive health. Let us reflect on the major lessons gathered throughout our journey as we review the key takeaways.

1. Recognizing Fertility Issues

Our journey began with a basic awareness of reproductive issues. Recognizing infertility as a shared experience, we divided between primary and secondary infertility, taking into account the various stories that occur within both realms.

2. The Role of Lifestyle and Nutrition in Fertility

The importance of diet and lifestyle emerged as a recurring subject. We investigated the critical significance of balanced nutrition, weight maintenance, and regular exercise in improving reproductive health. The link of physical health and the fertility journey emphasized the significance of a comprehensive strategy.

3. Insights into the Female Reproductive System and Menstrual Cycle

The first chapter delves into the deep aspects of the female reproductive system, revealing remarkable insights into the menstrual cycle's nuances. Our investigation focused on the stages, hormonal swings, and the amazing complexity that drives a woman's reproductive journey.

4. Dietary Influence on Fertility: Nutritional Guidelines

In Chapter 2, we moved our focus to the effect of diet on fertility, providing practical nutritional suggestions. Understanding the importance of necessary nutrients and following a fertility-friendly diet have become critical components in promoting reproductive health.

5. Lifestyle Factors: Stress Management and Physical Activity

Chapter 3 focused on lifestyle issues, with an emphasis on stress management and exercise. We investigated the complex relationship between stress and fertility, emphasizing the need of efficient coping techniques. Our investigation revealed the importance of exercise as a holistic strategy to supporting reproductive health.

6. Environmental Factors: Toxins and Creating a Fertility-Friendly Environment

Environmental factors take the stage in Chapter 4. We investigated the effects of pollutants on fertility and discussed ways for building a fertile environment. Recognizing the impact of extrinsic circumstances on reproductive health was an important part of our journey.

7. The Role of Supplements: Essential Nutrients and Supplements to Consider

Chapter 5 walked us through the role of supplements, highlighting important nutrients and reproductive supplements. Understanding the possible benefits of dietary supplements to enhance reproductive health provides a more nuanced view of the fertility landscape.

8. Men's Health and Fertility: Understanding Male Factors and Improvement Strategies

Our journey proceeded with Chapter 6, which focused on men's health and fertility. We learned about male characteristics that influence fertility and investigated ways for enhancing sperm quality. Recognizing the significance of male reproductive health emphasized the importance of a comprehensive approach to family formation.

9. Medical Interventions and Future Trends in Assisted Reproductive Technologies

Chapter 7 looked at medical interventions, including assisted reproductive technologies (ART) and future trends. Our investigation ranged from in vitro fertilization (IVF) to donor conception identity issues, global discrepancies in ART access, and the emotional and psychological aspects of fertility treatments.

10. Triumphs and Real-Life Experiences

We explored success stories in Chapter 8, appreciating the victories and real-life experiences of people and couples navigating the fertility path. These stories provided a vivid picture of perseverance, hope, and the varied roads to parenting, from overcoming obstacles and hurdles to discovering unexpected paths and embracing holistic approaches.

As we review these major points, it becomes clear that the fertility landscape is complex, multifaceted, and very personal. Our journey has exposed the challenges and accomplishments involved in the desire of forming a family, from understanding the physiological subtleties to embracing the emotional and psychological components.

May this summary serve as a compass, leading individuals and couples through the ever-changing terrain of fertility with insights, knowledge, and a sense of shared humanity. The fertility journey exemplifies human endurance, hope, and the incredible capacity for new beginnings.

Readers Empowered to Act: Navigating the Fertility Journey with Knowledge and Agency

As we get to the end of this enlightening look at fertility, the trip extends beyond the pages of knowledge to a call to action. A fundamental theme that runs through our comprehensive journey is empowering readers to take responsibility of their reproductive health, make informed decisions, and negotiate the intricacies of the fertility landscape with agency.

Knowledge as a Driver of Informed Decisions

You now have a lot of knowledge from our exploration to make informed decisions geared to your own situation. Understanding the complexities of the menstrual cycle, the impact of lifestyle on fertility, and the subtleties of medical interventions provides a solid foundation for decision-making. This knowledge is a powerful tool, allowing you to engage with healthcare experts in a proactive manner, ask informed questions, and actively participate in your fertility journey.

Options for Holistic Wellness and Lifestyle

The emphasis on holistic approaches, lifestyle changes, and nutrition serves as a roadmap for you as you strive to improve your reproductive health. Recognizing the relationship between physical well-being, mental health, and fertility enables you to develop balanced lifestyles that support your goals. Empowering yourself to act entails putting this knowledge into concrete activities, such as adding fertility-friendly foods, implementing stress management techniques, or including regular exercise into your wellness routine.

Using Informed Consent to Navigate Medical Interventions

Informed consent is the source of empowerment for persons contemplating or receiving medical interventions. You are encouraged to actively engage with healthcare providers, to inquire about potential risks and advantages, and to get familiar with the numerous options available. Whether you are considering fertility treatments, assisted reproductive technologies, or genetic testing, informed decision-making ensures that you have a say in your treatment choices.

Exploring New Routes and Accepting Diversity

Recognizing and appreciating the diversity inherent in the fertility process leads to empowerment. You are urged to consider alternative routes to parenthood, such as adoption, surrogacy, or unconventional family-building techniques. Understanding that success stories come in a variety of shapes and sizes develops a sense of inclusion, where you feel empowered to pick the routes that correspond with your values and objectives.

Reproductive Health Advocacy

Empowering oneself extends beyond your personal journey to reproductive health activism. Armed with knowledge, you may become an advocate for increased awareness, access to reproductive care, and the de-stigmatization of infertility conversations. By sharing your personal story, joining support groups, and engaging in open dialogues, you help to build a collective voice that promotes reproductive health as an essential component of overall well-being.

Emotional Well-Being and Mind-Body Connection

Given the importance of the mind-body connection in fertility, you are recommended to emphasize emotional well-being. In this sense, taking action is getting help when it is needed, whether through therapy, support groups, or mind-body activities like meditation and yoga. In order to navigate the emotional intricacies of the reproductive journey, it is necessary to cultivate emotional resilience.

Personalized Parenting Pathways

In the context of fertility, empowerment recognizes that there is no one-size-fits-all solution. You are invited to choose your own paths to motherhood that reflect your values, priorities, and unique circumstances. The ability to shape your journey is a vital component of the fertility narrative, whether you pursue fertility treatments, embrace alternative options, or choose for holistic wellbeing.

Finally, this call to action invites you to be an active participant in your fertility story. The knowledge gained is more than just information; it is a catalyst for empowerment. It's a compass that will help you navigate the complexity of the fertility landscape with agency, resilience, and optimism.

May this empowerment result in not only a successful fertility journey, but also a greater impact, influencing a culture in which conversations about reproductive health are open, supportive, and de-stigmatized. You can embark on your fertility journey with confidence, empowered to embrace the possibilities and create new beginnings, if you have knowledge, informed choices, and collective advocacy.

www.ingramcontent.com/pod-product-compliance
Lightning Source LLC
Chambersburg PA
CBHW070821250726

48662CB00003B/1036